Overcoming Common Problems

# Coping When Your Child Has Cerebral Palsy

JILL ECKERSLEY

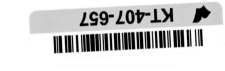

First published in Great Britain in 2009

Sheldon Press
36 Causton Street
London SW1P 4ST

*British Library Cataloguing-in-Publication Data*
A catalogue record for this book is available from the British Library

ISBN 978–1–84709–070–6

1 3 5 7 9 10 8 6 4 2

Typeset by Fakenham Photosetting Ltd, Fakenham, Norfolk
Printed in Great Britain by Ashford Colour Press

Produced on paper from sustainable forests

# Contents

# Acknowledgements and about the author

## Acknowledgements

I could not have written this book without the help of many healthcare professionals, notably Dr Richard Morton, Consultant Paediatrician at Derby Hospitals, Laura the physiotherapist, Jackie the dietician, the staff of the London Bobath Centre and Dr Linda Scotson.

As always, I would like to offer very special thanks to all the parents who have offered their opinions and expertise to benefit others, and to Robyn Carter of the website <www .special kidsintheuk.org>.

## About the author

Jill Eckersley is a freelance writer with many years' experience of writing on health topics. She is a regular contributor to women's and general-interest magazines, including *Bella*, *Women's Fitness*, *Slimming World* and other titles. *Coping with Snoring and Sleep Apnoea*, *Coping with Childhood Asthma*, *Coping with Dyspraxia*, *Coping with Childhood Allergies*, *Helping Children Cope with Anxiety*, *Every Women's Guide to Heart Health*, *Living with Eczema* and *Every Woman's Guide to Digestive Health*, eight books written by Jill for Sheldon Press, were all published between 2003 and 2008. She lives beside the Regent's Canal in north London with two cats.

# Introduction

Jess, aged three, is a sparky little girl with beautiful eyes. Teenager Gemma always has a big smile on her face and is a huge fan of the Harry Potter books. Nat is hoping to go to university after collecting ten GCSEs.

On the face of it these three children wouldn't seem to have much in common, but they do. All three are living with cerebral palsy, a common cause of childhood disability. Figures for the number of children affected range from one in 400 to one in 500, and in spite of better ante-natal care it seems that the figures have not changed very much. This is because cerebral palsy (cp) particularly affects babies born prematurely, and with more and more of the very tiniest premature babies surviving, that means more children with cp growing up. Twins and triplets are also at risk as many are premature. IVF and other fertility treatments mean that more and more multiple births are taking place. Research into the causes of, and treatments for, cerebral palsy is ongoing but doctors working in the field believe that the condition is unlikely to be eliminated completely in the near future.

'Having a child with cerebral palsy isn't the end of the world. It's just the beginning of a new one!' says one of the mothers interviewed for this book. If your baby or small child has just been diagnosed, however, it can feel rather as though your world has fallen apart and there will be many questions you want to ask. What in fact is cerebral palsy? What causes it? Was there anything you could have done to prevent it? How will it affect *your* baby . . . *your* toddler . . . *your* older child? What sort of life will your child have and how can you help your baby to ensure that he or she makes the most of it?

This book is intended to offer answers to some of those questions, with the help of 'experts' – both the doctors, teachers and other medical specialists who work with children with cerebral palsy, and the real experts, mums and dads who have to deal with the issues raised by having a child with cerebral palsy in the family on a daily basis.

Children with cerebral palsy are, first and foremost, *children*. They may need a little help – or quite a lot – to do the things their non-disabled brothers, sisters and friends take for granted, but at the end of the day they need what all children need – love, fun, security, a warm family life and the chance to fulfil their potential in every way possible.

How can you help your child with cerebral palsy do all that? Read on . . .

# 1

# What is cerebral palsy?

It is almost easier to say what cerebral palsy *isn't*. For instance, it's not a disease, or an illness, or something you can catch. It's a disorder, or impairment, following brain damage and affecting *movement* in one way or another. No two children with cp are affected in exactly the same way. For some, the difficulties are very mild and almost unnoticeable; for others, the impairment is extremely severe. The child may need to use a wheelchair and have little control over his or her movements.

When there is brain damage, the wrong messages are sent from the brain to the muscles.

There are three main types of cerebral palsy:

- *spastic* – the most common, affecting around 70 per cent of children with cp, where the child's muscles are stiff, tight and difficult to control;
- *athetoid* – which can affect posture and can cause unwanted movements;
- *ataxic* – which affects balance and can cause shaking movements as well as difficulties with speech in affected children.

It's possible for children to have more than one type of cerebral palsy at the same time. The word 'dystonic' is also used to describe children whose muscle tone varies between stiff and floppy. In addition, the condition is sometimes defined by the area of the body affected. 'Quadriplegia' means that all four of the child's limbs are affected. 'Hemiplegia' means that one side of the child's body is affected. 'Diplegia' means that the child's legs are affected more than other parts of the body. The effects can be mild, moderate or severe in any case.

Muscle tone plays a part in the diagnosis of cerebral palsy and can help doctors to decide which type of cp a child has, and therefore what kind of treatment might be most appropriate. It is

1

difficult to diagnose in a newborn, because newborn babies have a limited range of movements anyway. As the baby grows and develops, it becomes easier to see whether muscles are working normally. Normal muscle tone means the elasticity or tension in the muscles when a child is relaxed. All the muscles should then be able to move freely and easily. In children with cerebral palsy, the muscles might be unusually 'tight' or rigid, suggesting spastic cp. Or, alternatively, the muscles might be unusually floppy. Muscle tone can vary in an individual child, and may be affected by the effort involved as the child tries to move or speak. Muscle tone may also be affected by the child's mood – for instance, by tiredness, excitement or frustration.

Children with cerebral palsy may have other health problems – blindness, deafness, speech and language difficulties – and learning difficulties. Or they may not. The condition is as individual as children themselves are. About one third of children with cerebral palsy also have epilepsy – seizures caused by disruption to the normal electrical activity of the brain. Some children have digestive or respiratory problems, because the muscles in their digestive or respiratory systems don't respond in the way they should, so feeding and coping with everyday ailments like coughs and colds can be more difficult than they would otherwise be.

Because children with cerebral palsy may have trouble speaking clearly or controlling their movements or expressions, it's sometimes assumed that they all have learning difficulties. This is not necessarily so. Some children with cp have a high IQ, some have moderate or severe learning difficulties, but the majority are of average intelligence, just like children who don't have cp. It is a very individual condition.

## What causes cerebral palsy?

The condition is most usually caused by a failure of part of the brain to develop, because of events before, during or after birth.

The part of the brain involved is the cerebrum, which controls the muscles and is also involved in the development of communication skills, memory and the ability to learn. Better care of women in labour and birth in recent years has meant that only about one in ten cases are the result of complications at this stage. The vast majority, perhaps 80 per cent, are caused by factors which affect the developing baby in the womb.

These can include infections which the mother develops during pregnancy, for example rubella (German measles) or toxoplasmosis (an infection which can be spread by gardening, eating unwashed raw fruit and vegetables, or handling infected cat-litter). Infection can also be the result of cytomegalovirus, which can cause cerebral palsy and/or hearing problems. An active outbreak of herpes which develops *for the first time* when the baby is due can also be dangerous. A Caesarean section is usually recommended to avoid passing on the virus to the baby during a vaginal delivery. (Episodes of herpes which develop at other times during pregnancy pose little risk to your baby.)

In a very few cases, genetics may play a part. Very high or very low blood pressure in the mum-to-be, pelvic inflammatory disease, binge-drinking or the use of street drugs like cocaine can also result in damage to the developing baby's brain. Some cases of brain damage are the result of periventricular leukomalacia (PVL). This is defined as damage to the 'white matter', made up of nerve fibres, which is normally involved in directing communication between the 'grey matter' and the muscles. It is thought that this is a result of a reduction in the blood supply to the brain, which deprives it of oxygen.

A baby's brain is especially immature and therefore vulnerable during the first 30 weeks of pregnancy, when any mutating genes, infections or injuries may affect its development. Unborn babies can also suffer a stroke – bleeding in the brain itself – which can either deprive the brain of the blood it needs or damage the brain. It is not yet known why this happens although it might have some link with the way the afterbirth works, and researchers are looking at this possibility. The baby itself might have especially weak blood vessels.

In some cases, however, there is no apparent reason for a baby being born with cerebral palsy. It is also possible for an infection a previously healthy baby develops during infancy or early childhood, such as meningitis or encephalitis, to result in cerebral palsy.

## Can cerebral palsy be prevented? Who is at risk?

There are no absolute guarantees, although a healthy mum always has the best chance of producing a healthy baby! When you are planning to get pregnant, it's important to make sure that your vaccinations against diseases like rubella are up to date and that you take the best possible care of yourself. If you are a smoker, try and give up before embarking on a pregnancy. Ask your GP to refer you to local Stop Smoking clinics or contact the NHS 'Stop Smoking' helpline on 0800 169 0169.

Advice on 'safe drinking' levels during pregnancy tends to vary but it seems unlikely that the occasional beer or glass of wine will do any harm. If your pregnancy was unplanned and you are a regular drinker, don't panic, but do cut down – or, better still, stop drinking – as soon as you suspect you might be pregnant. A large recent study of more than 12,000 children and their mums by researchers at University College London found that drinking one or two alcohol units a week seemed to be safe. However, you might prefer to give up alcohol for the duration, just to be on the safe side, as Department of Health guidelines suggest. Binge-drinking is definitely out! As are illegal drugs of all types – it's just not worth risking your baby's life and health, not to mention your own.

There's plenty of advice available on healthy eating during pregnancy, though no particular diet is known to protect against cerebral palsy. A well-nourished mum with a strong immune system boosted by plenty of fruit and vegetables is most likely to have a healthy baby.

Although it isn't, at present, possible to diagnose cerebral palsy while the baby is still in the womb, it is vitally important for every mum-to-be to attend all her ante-natal appointments to be as sure as she can be that all is well. Cerebral palsy is linked to prematurity, especially extreme prematurity, and much of the current research into cp seems to be focused on preventing babies being born too soon. Those born before 28 weeks are especially at risk, and it seems that the more premature the baby, the greater the risk of some form of disability, including cerebral palsy. Ante-natal appointments can often reveal possible complications which might lead to premature birth with all its associated risks, so don't take chances. Attend all your appointments.

Very young mothers – aged 17 or younger – seem to be at slightly higher risk of having premature babies and the same applies to much older mothers – those over 35. As well as smoking, excess alcohol, drug use and social deprivation, all of which are associated with an increased risk of premature birth, women who have previously had a premature baby are also at higher risk.

## Premature babies and multiple births

The World Health Organization defines a 'premature' baby as one born before 37 weeks' gestation. Very low-birthweight babies (those weighing less than five and a half pounds, or 2.5 kilos) are most at risk of disability, About 7 per cent of UK babies – around 45,000 a year – are born weighing less than this and the percentage is higher in deprived areas. A tiny baby, born before any of its body systems are ready to cope with the outside world, is much more susceptible to developing brain damage.

One of the reasons the incidence of cerebral palsy in children is not falling, in spite of better ante-natal and maternity care, is that more very premature babies are now surviving. Special care baby units, or SCBUs, enable those born at just 25 weeks to have a roughly 50–50 chance of making it. Thirty years ago these babies would have died. Although the improvements in neonatal care are to be welcomed, it's also true that many of these very tiny babies grow up with some degree of impairment, including cerebral palsy.

IVF treatments for infertile couples also often result in twins, triplets or even higher 'multiple' births. These babies, too, are frequently premature and run the same risk of developing cerebral palsy. Twin pregnancies last, on average, 37 weeks, triplet pregnancies 33 weeks and quadruplet pregnancies 31 weeks. It is thought that 'multiples' are born early because the womb becomes over-stretched, although there is much we don't yet know about exactly why premature births occur. Clinics specializing in 'assisted conceptions' such as IVF are beginning to consider implanting fewer fertilized eggs, to reduce the risk of multiple pregnancies.

The government announced in September 2008 that it is hoping to reduce the numbers of multiple births after fertility treatment from the present 24 per cent to 10 per cent over three years.

That doesn't mean that every premature baby is likely to have long-term health problems or disabilities including cerebral palsy. Albert Einstein, Charles Darwin and Winston Churchill were all premature babies and all born long before the advantages of modern health care were available to mothers and babies! However, the risks are higher for tiny, very early babies.

A study of extremely premature babies born in the Nottingham area in a ten-month period in 1995 looked at survival rates and at the children's health when they were two and a half and six years old. These were among the very tiniest premature babies, born at under 26 weeks' gestation. Of 4,004 babies born, 1,200 were born alive and 39 per cent of these survived to go home. Eighteen per cent of these had some form of cerebral palsy when they were two and a half, and cp seemed to affect more boys than girls. By the age of six, 40 per cent had some form of disability, including cp in some cases. About half of those with cerebral palsy were seriously affected by it. A second, similar study of very premature babies was begun in 2006.

## Why are some babies born prematurely?

We simply don't know – or, at least, in about half of cases of premature birth the causes cannot be identified. Those causes which *are* known include those mentioned above – smoking or the use of other drugs during pregnancy, and multiple pregnancies. Some unlucky mums-to-be have an 'incompetent cervix' or neck of the womb, which means that the birth canal begins to open before term. It is sometimes possible for the cervix to be stitched to prevent this happening. Others have fibroids (non-malignant growths in the womb) or develop infections late in pregnancy. There may be problems with the placental blood supply. Some mums-to-be develop pregnancy-induced diabetes or obstetric cholestasis, a liver disorder. Kidney disease or blood-clotting disorders such as systemic lupus erythematosus (SLE) can also lead to premature birth, though they can sometimes be controlled by drugs.

Sometimes the doctors caring for a mother-to-be decide that her baby must be delivered early by Caesarean section in order to save its life or the mother's. Reasons for this can include

- a life-threatening condition called pre-eclampsia, revealed when the woman develops very high blood pressure and has high levels of protein in her urine;
- a kidney or urinary tract infection;
- diabetes in the mother;
- a condition called placenta praevia, when the placenta or after-birth is in the wrong part of the womb;
- placental abruption – when the placenta comes away from the wall of the womb;
- the baby becoming distressed or showing poor growth because of lack of oxygen or nourishment.

In many of the cases of premature birth in Britain every year, there is no obvious cause. Mums-to-be can give themselves and their babies the best chance of avoiding the risks of premature birth by taking care of themselves during pregnancy and, above all, by attending ante-natal appointments so that any potential problems can be spotted at an early stage.

## Multiple births and prematurity

With or without IVF or other assisted conception techniques, twin and multiple pregnancies often end in premature birth. US researchers claim that about 50 per cent of twins, 90 per cent of triplets and virtually all larger multiples, like quads, are born prematurely.

It's already known that multiple pregnancies carry higher health risks for both mother and baby. These include a condition called Twin to Twin Transfusion Syndrome (TTTS) which can lead to miscarriage or premature birth. Once thought to be very rare, it is now said to affect one in 1,000 pregnancies. TTTS only affects identical twin foetuses and happens when there is an abnormality of the placental blood vessels, resulting in an unbalanced flow of blood between the twins in the womb. The 'recipient' twin then has extra blood, which causes its heart to pump harder, and this can lead to heart failure or to disabilities such as cerebral palsy. The 'donor' twin has less blood and is smaller, though may be stronger as its heart has not had to work so hard. More information can be obtained from the Twin to Twin Transfusion Syndrome Association (contact details on p. 103).

## Finding out your baby has – or could have – cerebral palsy

It is always a shock to find out that your longed-for baby has, or might have, health problems. If the birth was especially traumatic or very premature, your first priority, as parents, is of course the baby's survival. Parents of newborns who are whisked off to special care units hardly have time to think beyond those first few anxious hours, days and weeks. Everyone's experience is different, as the following stories show.

Josh and his twin were born at 27 weeks with TTTS but no-one told us that he might have cerebral palsy, not in so many words – or maybe I just don't remember. When he was about six months old and obviously was not reaching the milestones other babies reach, I mentioned cerebral palsy to my doctor, who seemed relieved that I had brought the subject up! The boys are seven now and Josh is totally dependent. He has quadraplegic cerebral palsy. He has to be tube-fed; he can eat and swallow but his food has to be mashed up. He has epilepsy but only has fits if he's ill, and he is registered blind.

Matthew was born at 29 weeks, weighing only one pound nine ounces [0.7 kilo]. Because of his size and medical problems during his birth he had two bleeds into his brain. We were told he would never walk or talk. Now he is five, he does both – and very well, too. However, he does have ataxic cerebral palsy. Essentially he is a wonky walker who tires easily and uses a wheelchair for distance.

Jessica was five weeks old when the community nurse told us coldly and cruelly that she had cerebral palsy, though she had an MRI scan after her birth and it was suspected then. The doctors at the hospital didn't tell us, just vaguely said she might have a few problems. We were given a heap of handouts from SCOPE and that was it. We have found everything else out ourselves, mainly from the Special Kids in the UK online forum [<www.specialkidsintheuk.org>] which has been an invaluable support network.

I knew from Darcey's birth that there was something wrong. She was born late, at 43 weeks, but only weighed four pounds [1.8 kilos], and the birth was very traumatic. Her development was slow and she had digestive problems, but it wasn't until she had a brain scan at a year old that I was given a diagnosis of cerebral palsy. She is almost two now, and although her arms and legs don't work properly she can roll over and is beginning to talk.

Iain was almost full term but was quite small at five and a half pounds [2.5 kilos]. I had an emergency Caesarian as he was becoming distressed. Just after he was born he developed a chest infection and very low blood sugar. We were not given a diagnosis until he was ten months old. At the time it was made light of. We were given the impression that, with some physio, he would be fine. In fact he has no mobility at all and can only use his left hand. He has good head control, can speak and uses a motorized wheelchair. We still don't know what actually caused the cerebral palsy.

Dr Richard Morton is Consultant Paediatrician at Derby Hospitals and has a special interest in children with disabilities, including cerebral palsy. He and his team regularly have to tell new parents that their child may have the condition and, he says, they try to be as factual as possible while remaining sensitive and sympathetic.

Many parents already have an inkling there is something wrong, because the baby was born pre-term or very small, there was an infection or the baby had breathing or heart problems at birth, for example. In other cases cerebral palsy will not be detected until the baby is six months old, perhaps because parents have noticed that their baby is not reaching the normal milestones for her age.

I would say that more than half of the parents I work with know their baby is at risk of cp because it was premature or there were difficulties around the birth.

Mild or moderate cerebral palsy can be quite hard to diagnose until a baby is three to five months old. A severely affected baby may have an irritable cry, may feed only with difficulty, may seem to have abnormal, jerky movements or perhaps very little movement.

Other babies seem all right at first but simply don't reach their milestones. By about five months, for instance, a baby should be using both its hands and not just one. A baby with cerebral palsy might have very stiff limbs or be unable to sit up. Or it might have digestive problems, have trouble feeding or be sick a lot. My message for parents would be: if there is something that worries you, discuss it, first with your health visitor or GP and if necessary with a specialist. Slow development should be looked into, rather than assuming that the baby will 'grow out of it'.

It isn't easy to live with an uncertain diagnosis, but at this stage it can be hard to know for sure whether the baby does have cerebral palsy, and if it does, how mildly or severely it might be affected in the future.

'The older the child gets the easier it is to predict,' says Dr Morton.

By the time the baby is a year old we can tell if it will be severely affected. By the age of two, we should be able to tell the parents if their child will be able to walk and talk. One predictor is that if the child is unable to sit by the age of two, it's unlikely that he will be able to walk without help.

When we tell parents their child has cp, we also tell them that although there is nothing we can do to change the brain function itself – in other words, cure the cerebral palsy – there is a lot we can do to improve quality of life. There are therapies, medicines, surgical treatments and technological developments which can help. Good parenting is terribly important too; parents can work with physios, occupational and speech and language therapists, as well as paediatricians – and above all, learn to love their children and value them as they are!

# 2

# Cerebral palsy and your baby

Perhaps the hardest issue for parents of newborns to face is uncertainty. First of all, of course, is the uncertainty about whether or not your premature or sick newborn will even survive. Then there is the uncertainty about his or her future. You may be told straight away that there is a chance your baby may have suffered brain damage, or you may not. If the birth was perfectly normal and straightforward you may not have any idea that your baby has cerebral palsy until he or she doesn't reach the normal baby milestones – lifting the head, rolling over, sitting up, crawling, walking and so on. There are shocks, too, if your baby develops cerebral palsy as the result of a serious illness like meningitis and you are suddenly faced with the prospect of looking after a disabled child who, before the illness, had always seemed perfectly healthy.

It can't be emphasized enough that cerebral palsy is a highly individual condition and – rather like children who don't have any disability – children with this condition all develop in their own time and in their own way.

Understandably, most parents would prefer to know straight away what the future holds, but unfortunately it just isn't possible for even the experts to tell you that. As we saw in the last chapter, some health professionals don't mention it at this early stage; others offer a gloomier prognosis than turns out to be the case. It is always a fine line between giving parents false hope and no hope at all.

In any case, there is a lot to get used to and it will take time for you to adjust to the new reality. This is where the support of friends and family, and especially of other parents who know what you are going through, can be invaluable. See pages 98–103 for contact details for organizations like SCOPE, Bliss and online parents' support groups. SCOPE, for example, runs Face2Face projects in some areas of the country, where parents who have a child with cerebral palsy befriend and support others.

## If your baby needs special care

A special care baby unit or SCBU can be a frightening place even when you know that it is also the safest place for your premature or sick newborn to be. While the other mums on the maternity ward have their healthy babies with them for at least some of the time, yours is some distance away. You don't have the same opportunities to get to know, bond with and cuddle the new arrival. If your baby has particular problems he or she may even need to be transferred to another hospital with an intensive-care SCBU where there are specialist staff and facilities.

This is an anxious time for you and you might well experience a feeling of complete unreality. Nothing has turned out the way you expected or planned. It is quite normal to wonder whether the baby is really yours. You might feel desperately protective and concerned that there seems to be so little you can do for him or her. You will certainly feel afraid of what might happen, and may be shocked when you do visit the SCBU and see your newborn in a special cot or incubator.

Very premature or sick babies need to be in a temperature-controlled environment. They need help to fight off possible infections. They often need help with breathing as their lungs may not be sufficiently developed for them to breathe unaided, so they are attached to a ventilator. They will probably have to be tube- or drip-fed until they have developed enough to feed normally.

You may be shocked at your baby's appearance – not only tiny, fragile and terribly vulnerable, but also thin, without the plump, rounded look of a healthy newborn, and with a red or even hairy skin.

All these reactions are absolutely normal. Don't be afraid to ask the staff of the SCBU what is happening to and around your baby. They are specially trained to care for very tiny and sick babies and will be able to reassure you and explain what all the technology is used for.

Your baby's incubator is basically a temperature-controlled, see-through cabinet supplied with warm air and oxygen to help the baby to breathe. Some of the wires you see attached to your baby's skin are connected to monitors which check breathing, heart rate and temperature 24/7. Feeding tubes may be passed through the baby's nostrils or directly into the stomach. Breast milk is the best food for your baby and the nurses will show you how you can express your own breast milk for him or her. Expressing breast milk regularly will help your body to establish its own milk supply, as will making sure you get enough rest and are well nourished yourself. Alternatively, your baby can be fed from a 'milk bank'.

The fact that your baby is in special care and being looked after by trained professionals doesn't mean that you are not needed or that you can't play any part in his or her care. Far from it. Tiny and sick babies need all the love and care you can give them. The SCBU nurses will show you how you can touch and stroke your baby through the portholes in the incubator. Your baby will recognize your voice, so talk and sing to him or her as much as you can and encourage your partner to do the same.

When your baby is well enough to come out of the incubator for a cuddle it's a special moment, but it can also be terrifying because he or she seems so tiny and fragile.

'The little bundle seemed more blanket than baby. It was wonderful to be able to hold her at last, but terrifying too because she was still so tiny. When she was born, she looked like a boiled monkey, to be honest,' says one mum, describing her two-months-premature daughter.

Some SCBUs recommend what is known as 'kangaroo care', where both Mum and Dad are encouraged to give the baby skin-to-skin contact. It's said that babies cuddled in this way cry less, sleep better and have more oxygen in their blood. Babies also need to get used to their mum's individual smell, so take every opportunity you can to cuddle your baby while he or she is in special care. The nurses will help you to get involved with the caring routines – feeding, changing and washing – and the more you do this, the more confident you will feel when your baby is eventually well enough to leave hospital and come home.

If your baby has to spend weeks or months in hospital it is important for both of you – and not forgetting Dad – to spend as much time as you can together.

## Epilepsy

About a third of babies and children with cerebral palsy also have epilepsy. Epileptic seizures (which used to be known as 'fits') are caused by a sudden burst of electrical activity in the brain. Seizures in tiny babies are sometimes difficult to recognize and/or diagnose, as it is not always obvious what is happening. A seizure may only cause altered breathing patterns and some eyelid movement, or it may result in unusual movement of the baby's arms or legs, or 'jerking' motions of the limbs or body.

If your baby's carers suspect that seizures have occurred, he or she will be referred for an electroencephalogram (EEG), which can detect the most subtle of problems if interpreted by a paediatric EEG specialist. A range of medication is available for the treatment of seizures, even in infants. However, it can be difficult for doctors to say whether or not the seizures will continue or how they might affect your baby's future development.

## At home with your baby

Your baby won't be allowed home until the staff of the SCBU and other specialists are sure that he or she can cope outside the controlled environment that is 'special care'. The baby will still look small and fragile when he or she does come home with you. Especially for first-time parents, it can feel overwhelming to realize that *you* are now responsible for this delicate little creature. A question-mark over your baby's current health or future prognosis is likely to leave you feeling even more worried.

Try to create as relaxed and comfortable a home for the newcomer as you can. Accept all the help you are offered by friends and family. You will also be encouraged to stay in touch with the SCBU staff and to call up if there are any questions. Hopefully by this time you will have some experience of caring for your baby, learned while he or she was still in special care.

As explained in the previous chapter, it's not always possible to tell whether the baby has cerebral palsy at this early stage. Even if you are given the diagnosis or it is suggested, it's unlikely that the doctors caring for your baby will know for sure just what the future holds and whether he or she is likely to be mildly, moderately or severely affected.

Like all new parents, you will watch your baby's development with fascination – and with some apprehension. It's all part of getting to know the newcomer, noting how she reacts to you and to the world around her, what she likes, what she doesn't like. Whether your baby has cp or not, she needs the same loving care. As well as practical care – feeding, washing, changing – your baby needs you to talk to her, sing to her, stroke and cuddle her.

### Baby massage

Baby massage is traditional in many cultures and is increasing in popularity here. It is said to be a good way to bond with your new baby and may also help with sleep and digestive problems. It is also a stress-reliever for anxious new mums, and may even help with post-natal depression.

You can find out more about baby massage from clinics, including complementary health clinics, and from the National Childbirth Trust (contact details on p. 100). It is sometimes said that it's better to wait until after your baby's first vaccinations to begin massage. Other experts recommend starting as soon as possible, even if your baby was premature and/or seems delicate. For babies at risk of disability, massage may help by improving muscle tone and stimulating growth hormones. Obviously, if your baby seems uncomfortable or appears not to like gentle stroking, then don't continue. It's always as well to check with your health visitor, paediatrician or the nurses who cared for your baby in SCBU.

Baby massage can include a lot of different techniques such as 'the open book', 'milking' and 'rolling' as well as straightforward stroking. Experiment to find out what your baby especially enjoys. If you are concerned about how firm a massage should be on a tiny baby, place your finger on your closed eyelid and stop when it begins to feel uncomfortable. That's the recommended level of pressure when massaging a very small baby. Movements can be a little firmer when your baby is older.

The website <www.netmums.com> gives advice on baby massage.

It suggests you choose a time of day when both you and your baby are relaxed, not tired, and at least half an hour after a feed. Make sure the room is warm. Dim lights and soft music can also increase the relaxing atmosphere. Lie your baby on an old towel or muslin on a changing mat, without clothes or a nappy, and make eye contact with him or her.

Oil your hands and rub them together to warm them. Use either baby oil or a non-fragranced oil such as grapeseed. Take a look at the Weleda range of baby products, which are made from 100 per cent natural ingredients. Their Calendula Oil is recommended for baby massage.

Then try some gentle strokes from your baby's shoulders to her feet, repeating each movement six times. Then similar gentle strokes from her chest outward and down her arms. You can also circle your fingertips clockwise over her tummy. Then shoulders-to-feet again, followed by gentle strokes down each thigh, repeated six times. If she is happy to lie on her tummy you can turn her over to stroke down her back and legs, using more oil if required. To end the session, hold your warmed hands at the base of her back or on her shoulders for a few moments.

Remove any excess oil with a towel or muslin and dress her again. The whole experience should be done slowly, gently and without any rush so that both of you are completely comfortable and relaxed.

## Who can help?

There are many different health professionals who can offer advice on caring for new babies with possible disabilities. Apart from the midwives, SCBU staff and the paediatrician you saw when your baby was still in hospital, your GP and health visitor will play a part in her care in the early days and weeks. She may then be referred for further help from a physiotherapist, occupational therapist (OT), speech and language therapist and even a dietician, depending on the difficulties which arrive as she grows and develops. A 'key worker' may be appointed to co-ordinate all the professional help. In the very early days your key worker will probably be your health visitor; later, a social worker will take over if needed.

## Physiotherapy and your baby

Physiotherapists are experts in body movement and understand how muscles and joints work. A physio may be brought in to help with diagnosis, to assess your baby's condition and discover whether she does have cerebral palsy. If there are concerns about your baby's development, either because she was premature, because the birth was difficult or because she doesn't seem to be reaching her milestones at her developmental checks, then she may be referred to a physiotherapist.

'Cerebral palsy can cause a wide spectrum of problems, from the very subtle to the highly complex,' says Laura, a Liverpool-based physiotherapist who has worked with children and families for 25 years.

> We always like to see children earlier, rather than later. We usually see babies from about eight months old, by which time we would expect a baby to be sitting up, although some children are referred to us at two and a half or three. We start the assessment as soon as the child is referred to us and give the parents simple advice on activities and positioning, based on their baby's individual needs.
>
> We will always look at what the baby can do, how she moves, and the quality of the movement, then identify the reasons why she can't move in the way we would expect. We feel the baby to assess her muscle tone, whether it is stiff or floppy or seems normal. We look at things like the baby's head control, whether she can move her head to follow the movement of a toy, whether she can move both hands to her mouth, kick her legs, reach for her knees and feet, or lift her head up if she is lying on her tummy.

Based on these observations, physios like Laura can make suggestions that will help you to help your baby to move more easily. At this young age, this involves games and activities rather than formal 'physiotherapy', all aimed at promoting your baby's development and normalizing muscle tone.

Especially if you are first-time parents, it can be difficult to tell whether any problems your baby might have are linked to cerebral palsy or not. Some babies are 'difficult' feeders, some are poor sleepers, some are livelier and more mobile than others at an earlier age, even when they don't have health problems. It's easier said than done, but do try not to worry too much. Baby development is not a competition!

## If your baby has problems feeding

Cerebral palsy can affect the sucking reflex, as it can affect other kinds of movement, so your baby may not feed easily whether breast- or bottle-fed. If you are breast-feeding, make sure you are eating well and resting as much as possible. If your baby's muscles are especially stiff or especially floppy, she will need a lot of support for her head and back. It may take time to establish a feeding position which suits you both. You could try holding your baby under your arm, supporting her chin and jaw with the same hand you use to support your breast.

Ask for advice from your midwife or health visitor, who can help you make sure that your baby has latched on to your breast correctly. If she finds it especially difficult, 'special needs feeders' are available to make it easier for her and for you. You'll need to be patient and remember that the cuddling and the skin-to-skin contact involved in feeding is as important to your baby as the actual nursing. Like any new mum you may experience difficulties too, such as sore, cracked nipples, or be worried that your baby is not getting enough milk. Discuss any worries like this with your health visitor, or contact breastfeeding experts like the La Leche League (contact details on p. 100).

## Speech and language therapy and your baby

It may surprise you to know that speech and language therapists can also give advice on feeding problems. As well as working on children's speech and language, they know how mouths, tongues and the swallowing reflex *should* work, and how to help little ones who have difficulties with these basic skills.

Says Katie Price of the Neurodisability Service at Great Ormond Street Hospital in London, 'Our role for children with cerebral palsy includes assessment, diagnosis and management of all aspects of safe and effective nutrition, as well as speech development, understanding and use of language.'

It is quite common for babies with cerebral palsy to suffer from gastric reflux, a condition where the stomach contents flow back into the oesophagus or gullet because the valve between the two is too weak to prevent this happening. Babies with reflux may refuse to feed or find swallowing difficult, suffer from excessive wind, gag or choke or vomit a lot, experience poor weight gain, and even have breathing difficulties.

If your baby is diagnosed with reflux, it can help to position her in such a way that gravity prevents the feeds from being regurgitated, which means in a more upright position. You can feed her while standing up or walking around with her in a sling, or with *you* lying back against a pile of pillows and your baby with her face to your breast. It can also help to keep her upright for a time after each feed.

You may also be advised to place your baby's cot at an angle, that is, raised up at one end, and to offer frequent, small feeds.

## Weaning your baby

Breast milk is the ideal food for your baby until she is around six months old. Introducing your baby to solid food can pose particular problems if she has cerebral palsy. She may have limited control over the muscles of her head, face and neck, and over the movement of her tongue, lips and jaw, and this will affect her ability to chew, drink and swallow.

Helping your baby learn to cope with different foods should be a team effort, focusing on her individual needs. She might benefit from a specialized chair which helps her to sit upright and holds her head firmly; adapted cups and spoons; and food prepared in an appropriate way, so that she can learn to explore different tastes and textures like any other child.

As mentioned above, a speech and language therapist, an occupational therapist or a dietician may be the best person to advise you. With practice, you can learn what type of diet or texture of food suits your baby best – for example, thick liquids may be easier to control than water or juice. You could try offering very small amounts of pureed food, widening the teat in a bottle to enable something like porridge or yoghourt to be eaten, or if your baby has little control over her tongue, you could try to place food at the side of her mouth.

Some children will always have to be tube-fed via a naso-gastric tube, or may have a gastrostomy. This is a surgical opening into the stomach, which allows a feeding device to be inserted. Then the child can be fed directly into the stomach and the mouth and throat are not involved. A child who has difficulty chewing or swallowing is at risk of choking and breathing in food, which can lead to infections such as pneumonia, so if your baby finds it hard to cope with solids a gastrostomy may be recommended. Unlike a naso-gastric tube, it isn't obvious as it can be hidden under clothes. Different kinds of feeding devices are available and your doctor will explain which is best for your child. You will then be shown how to manage the appliance, and a sterile liquid which is a complete food in concentrated form will be recommended by your paediatric dietician. A gastrostomy can be reversed at a later date if it is felt that your child will be able to manage without it.

Rosemary's daughter Gemma found sucking and feeding very difficult and had a gastrostomy when she was 15 months old.

> Before that, feeding was a real struggle and she just didn't put on weight even though I poured yoghourt – which seemed to be all she could tolerate – down her. After she had the tube in her stomach we never looked back and she has been fed like that ever since. She now has a specially prescribed liquid diet because she can't co-ordinate her muscles enough to swallow.
>
> Gemma's personality seemed to change as soon as her nutrition was sorted out. Before that she had just cried all the time and I was rarely able to put her down. Once she was properly nourished she also started sleeping through the night for the first time.

Children with cerebral palsy who have feeding problems may be referred to specialized feeding clinics where they will be assessed by a paediatric dietician and sometimes a gastro-enterologist. It is reassuring to know that, given a personally tailored nutrition programme containing the right number of calories, your baby will grow and develop without risk of becoming either under-nourished or overweight.

## If your baby doesn't sleep

It can be hard to tell whether your baby is a poor sleeper, like many others, or if his or her sleep patterns are related to the cerebral palsy. SCOPE claims that children with cp *are* more likely to have sleep problems, and have a special section of their website devoted to 'Sleep Solutions'. Specially adapted cognitive or behavioural techniques are recommended. For contact details, see p. 101. The Scotson Technique, which is a therapy aimed at improving breathing techniques in children with cerebral palsy (see p. 83), can also be effective in improving sleep patterns.

Disturbed sleep can be caused by reflux and trapped wind making the baby feel uncomfortable, or by chronic pain in the baby's stiff muscles. Many parents report that their babies sleep better when cuddled.

Having a baby with a disability need not mean endless sleepless nights, however. Like all babies, those with cp respond best to consistent 'sleep cues' and a regular, soothing bedtime routine. Any changes, for instance cutting out a night-time feed, should be introduced gently and gradually. A multi-sensory approach can help. When putting your baby to bed, dim the light, draw the curtains, give her a warm bath and perhaps a brief massage, followed by gentle rocking, singing and a final cuddle before putting her to bed. Even the same bath oil or cream with a familiar scent of lavender can help to induce sleep.

## The 'alternative' approach

If your baby has a disability it is, of course, tempting to try *anything* that you think might help, and the advent of the Internet means that it is much simpler than it used to be to research alternative approaches to care. Be careful, though, as many so-called 'therapies' are unregulated and untested. Having said that, although no therapy will 'cure' cerebral palsy, some complementary treatments can be helpful, as consultant paediatrician Dr Richard Morton acknowledges.

What parents need is good professionals that they can trust. Parents should discuss all the possibilities and all the treatments with their care team. Complementary therapies can sometimes reduce the impact of cerebral palsy though they can't change the brain function itself. The help available on the NHS is very good, it's just that there isn't enough of it in every area and many therapists have full caseloads!

As an example, cranial osteopathy is recommended by many parents and Dr Morton agrees that it can be very soothing.

Osteopathy is a system of diagnosis and treatment which aims to restore the body to a state of balance and harmony. Cranial osteopathy is a subtle form of treatment which can encourage the release of stresses and tensions throughout the body, including the head. The theory is that birth itself can causes stresses that affect babies' heads. A cranial osteopath will gently manipulate the bones of the head and face to improve the circulation in the cerebro-spinal fluid which surrounds the brain. Although there is little conventional scientific evidence that it works, and no reputable practitioner would claim that it cures cerebral palsy, it does seem to help some babies' physical comfort, co-ordination and development. Parents often say that they notice a difference in their babies' crying, colic, sleeping and feeding difficulties after a session or sessions. You do, of course, need to be sure that the person you are consulting is qualified and experienced.

Annie, mum of three-year-old Jessica, who is severely physically disabled and cannot yet walk or talk, says she cannot praise her cranial osteopath enough.

'We see her once a fortnight and she is our saviour!' she says simply.

Gemma saw a cranial osteopath every week from the age of four months to three years and her mum also said it made a huge difference.

'She would cry all the way there but it calmed and relaxed her and she slept all the way home,' she says. 'It was a huge help for Gemma and for us.'

Activities such as baby yoga or mum-and-baby swimming classes may also be appropriate for a baby with cerebral palsy. Splashing around in warm water can be relaxing as well as stimulating and can help with muscle co-ordination and development.

# 3

# The early years

As your child grows and develops, some of the uncertainties about how he or she will be affected by cerebral palsy should begin to disappear.

'The older a child is, the better we, as professionals, can predict whether or not they actually have cerebral palsy, and if they do, how they will be affected,' says Dr Morton, Consultant Paediatrician at Derby Hospitals.

> By the time a baby is a year old it is usually obvious if she has severe cp, and by the age of two we should be able to tell whether she will be able to walk and talk. There are some predictors. For example, if a child cannot sit up by the age of two, it's unlikely he or she will be able to walk without help. Parents really don't need to spend their time or their money trying to help their child learn to do something that just isn't possible.
>
> Having said, that, good parenting is terribly important so that children can be helped to learn what they *can* do. Physiotherapists, OTs and speech and language therapists can help by directing the parents first.

Empowering families so that they are given the skills and confidence to manage their child's condition is very important, agrees physiotherapist Laura from Liverpool. 'We may start by helping a baby in its pram or on Mum's knee and then start to see the family on a regular basis, depending on the child's needs,' she says.

> At my own centre we stay with the family till the child is old enough for nursery, then transfer responsibility to a community physiotherapist. As long as there is an identified need, we are there to help. The amount of intervention needed can vary at different stages of a child's life. They may need more help during growth spurts, for instance, and there is usually a more formulated programme of activities for older children.

The main problem for children with cp is weakened muscles, so from the age of about four or five we will introduce a strengthening programme. With younger children we may focus on improving their environment and, when they are older, suggesting equipment like a stationary bike that they can use. We always look first at what the child is doing, find out why, and work out what we can do to help.

That may involve what are known as AFOs (ankle-foot orthoses) or splints, or equipment to help the child stand, sit or walk more easily, for instance a walking or standing frame. Occupational therapists come in at the same time, looking at the child's fine motor skills and recommending things like feeding equipment or supportive chairs.

Then there's the question of mobility, which could mean buggy adaptations or the use of a wheelchair as the child grows.

By this time, the team caring for your child should be well established and able to advise you on the kind of practical help with sitting, standing, feeding and walking which is required – and available. The government's SureStart programme is aimed at giving every child – including those with disabilities – the best possible start in life. By 2010, there should be 3,500 Children's Centres in the UK, bringing together early education, health, childcare and family support.

It is also important to remember that not *every* problem that comes up is a result of your child's cerebral palsy! A 'terrible two' is a 'terrible two', and although your child may experience extra frustration because he can't manage to do what some of his peers can, temper tantrums, refusal to eat or to sleep at night might just be because he is a feisty, stroppy toddler testing out his will-power on Mum and Dad!

As Laura says,

Just like any other children, those with cerebral palsy have to learn to play, occupy themselves in a high chair, and not demand attention all the time. Although you always need to be mindful of the implications of the cp, your child needs to learn that her parents are still in charge. Children with cp can have the same behaviour issues as other children. Parents learn to tell whether their child is genuinely in pain, upset or distressed or simply being difficult!

## Mobility aids

However much, or little, movement your child has, he needs to be encouraged to explore the world around him, his toys and his own personal space as far as he is able. Your physio or OT will have plenty of opportunities to observe your child and will recommend suitable help. The Disabled Living Foundation (contact details on p. 99) offers free and impartial advice on daily living equipment, mobility equipment and play equipment and can also provide a list of suppliers. It can help to talk to other parents about the type of equipment they have found helpful, although you always have to bear in mind children's varying needs. Positioning your child correctly can make a huge difference to his experience of the world as well as his health. You could consider

- a standing frame: different types are available and they are intended to help a child stand upright, stretch the muscles, cope with standing for longer periods and strengthen the muscles in the child's neck and body;
- a buggy: a specialized buggy will be lighter in weight than a wheelchair but will still need to be pushed;
- a wheelchair: both electric and manual chairs can be suitable for children from about 18 months onwards. Electrically powered indoor/outdoor chairs (EPIOCs) can be provided by the NHS without any age restriction as long as
  - the child is unable to propel a manual wheelchair;
  - having a powered chair will improve his or her quality of life;
  - he or she is able to handle it safely;
- a walking frame: this will provide extra stability and support for a child who can stand but needs some help in walking or moving around.

It's worth remembering, too, that ordinary play equipment can be therapeutic and enjoyable for your child to touch, feel, play with or roll around in or on!

## Mealtimes

The team caring for your child from earliest babyhood can offer help right through the early years. Play and exercise, appropriate equipment, speech therapy and the right diet can combine to help your child grow and develop healthily in spite of the cp. Nutrition is just as important for children with cerebral palsy as it is for any other children, although as they grow feeding can still pose problems, as Manchester-based dietician Jackie explains.

> For some children feeding is not an issue, but for others it can be a problem right from the start. Children are usually referred to me and to speech and language therapists via a consultant paediatrician or a paediatric neurologist. Once a family is referred to us, we offer ongoing help. This may also involve a physio and an OT, because the right seating, and the right positioning, can make all the difference to a child's ability to eat. It is very much a team approach.
>
> As children grow their calorie requirements obviously increase, but sometimes children with cp simply can't eat *enough* to provide all the nourishment they need. I can advise on how to feed a child to make sure that what she *does* eat is as nourishing as possible. Sometimes this means giving advice on the consistency of food, whether the child can manage thick liquids only, or pureed solids. Sometimes I recommend specially formulated supplementary foods or drinks with a high vitamin and protein content. As the child grows and her requirements change, different products may become more appropriate.
>
> Children with cp do sometimes have digestive problems. A child who is not mobile, and is unable to exercise, may be unable to tolerate large volumes of food and her stomach may be slow to empty. If her intake is limited this can contribute to constipation, and there are fibre-added products I may recommend. A child who spends a lot of time curled up in a chair or bed may suffer from gut motility problems, which is why the right seating and positioning is so important. Medication can also affect gut health.

## Dribbling

When your child is able to cope with a more solid diet it can become obvious that he is dribbling, or drooling. Drooling can lead to practical problems like sore skin around the mouth and throat, infections, dehydration or choking. About a third of children with cerebral palsy experience problems with drooling, which are often the result of swallowing difficulties or an inability to move saliva to the back of the throat to be swallowed, because of poor muscle control. Children who find it hard to close their mouths fully, who breathe through their mouths or have problems controlling the movement of their heads also tend to drool. With some children it happens more when they are excited or lose concentration.

If your child drools a lot he will benefit from an ear, nose and throat (ENT) examination to discover exactly why this is happening. Solutions are available ranging from simple 'rewards' offered when he manages to swallow to specially devised mouth exercises, Botox or, as a last resort, surgery to remove the salivary gland. A discussion with the ENT specialist and/or your speech and language therapist can help you to decide on the best solution for your child. In the meantime, it's important to keep his mouth, chin and throat as clean and dry as possible.

## Toilet training

Children without disabilities usually begin to understand what their potty is for between the ages of two and three years. It does vary, however, and there's no special advantage to the child in being toilet-trained very young, even though most parents are understandably glad to see the end of the nappy era!

Children with cerebral palsy tend to be older before they are ready to use a potty or the toilet. Some, of course, never master it, although it is helpful for a child's self-confidence if he or she can manage it. If your child's muscle control is very poor and he has little speech, ask your GP or paediatrician if they think he is able to tell when he needs to go, or if he is able to control the necessary muscles. If the answer is 'no', contact the various continence advisory services (contact details on p. 99) for help and advice on meeting his toileting and personal care needs.

If you are thinking of toilet training your child, SCOPE has a checklist which will help you work out whether he is ready to learn. For instance:

- Can he stay dry for an hour or more?
- Does he know what a potty or the toilet is for?
- Is he aware when his nappy is wet or soiled?
- Is his poo normal?
- Can he sit without support?
- Does he imitate what others do?
- Can he concentrate for five minutes or longer?
- Does he understand simple questions and can he indicate simple needs?

If the answer to most of these questions is 'yes', then by all means try toilet training him. Use the same method as you would with any toddler – no fuss about accidents and lots of praise when he manages to perform or ask for his potty. You can make it easier for yourself by watching his daily habits – does he tend to fill his nappy at a particular time, for instance after meals or first thing in the morning? That could be a good time to sit him on the potty. Some parents say that summertime, when the child is likely to be wearing fewer clothes, is an easier time to toilet train. On a warm sunny day a child can be left without pants or a nappy.

Make sure the potty you choose is comfortable and supportive, especially if your child has problems sitting or needs support. Ask advice from your OT if he needs special equipment. Even a child with little speech can often learn to sign, point, fidget or cry when he needs to go. Keep the potty where he can see it, and if your child has other carers, from grandparents to childminders, do tell them to look out for his signs or signals.

Like all parents you will need to be patient. Learning to use a potty doesn't happen overnight and may take a child with cp that bit longer. If he doesn't seem to be getting the idea at all, then leave it for a few weeks and try again.

Some children with cerebral palsy seem to suffer disproportionately from constipation, sometimes because of a limited diet or because their digestive system doesn't work as efficiently as it might. This can make toilet training difficult as the child begins to associate the potty or toilet with discomfort, pain and straining. If this is the case with your child, get advice from your GP about dealing with the constipation. A change in diet, as mentioned above, or a gentle laxative such as Lactulose may be prescribed to help. Some parents find that gently massaging the child's stomach can help to get things moving.

At some point your child may feel confident enough to progress from potty to toilet. Many children, including those without any disability, find this frightening. They may feel insecure sitting there without support or be afraid they will fall in and be flushed away. Lots of reassurance can help, plus praise for being a 'big boy' and using the toilet just like Mummy and Daddy.

Progress may well be slow, but if it doesn't seem to be happening at all or your child is becoming distressed, you could contact an organization called ERIC (which stands for Education and Resources for Improving Childhood Continence) – contact details are on p. 99. SCOPE and Contact a Family also have helpful tips on toilet training and related issues.

## Learning to communicate

More than 1.2 million children and young people in the UK have a communication impairment, and many of these are the result of cerebral palsy. If the muscles around your child's mouth and throat don't work very well, he will have problems learning to speak just as he has problems feeding. Not being able to speak does not, however, mean that your child can't communicate at all. Children with cerebral palsy can learn to use their hands, eye contact, body language, laughing and crying to let you know exactly what they are trying to say. With skilled help from a speech and language therapist, many or all of these skills can be mastered.

Learning to communicate is not necessarily about 'mouth exercises', which have actually not been found very effective. These days, helping children with communication difficulties is more about what are known as Augmentative and Alternative Communication (AAC) systems – which can include eye pointing, gesture, signing, using symbol or word boards or electronic speech devices. Voice output devices (VODs) are portable computers which 'talk' when they are activated. They can be operated by push-buttons, a switch with a scanner or a head-pointer, or by an infra-red system.

Much help is available, and speech and language therapists say that early intervention can be the key to helping your child make himself understood.

## If your child has epilepsy . . .

As already explained in the previous chapter, it is thought that about a third of children with cerebral palsy also have epilepsy. There are many different kinds of epileptic seizures, depending on exactly which part of the brain is affected. Some are almost unnoticeable – your child may just seem to be 'not quite there' for a few moments. Others – the classic *grand mal* seizure – can appear more frightening, with the child losing consciousness, perhaps falling, having convulsions and possibly losing bowel or bladder control. There are other types of seizures known as 'partial seizures' which can cause symptoms such as muscle spasms without loss of consciousness.

Anti-epilepsy drugs such as sodium valproate are very effective at controlling epileptic seizures, though it may take a little time to find a suitable drug and ensure that the dosage is right for your child. Like all drugs, these can have side effects which need to be monitored. Once your child's medication is adjusted for him, seizures are likely to be few and far between, if they happen at all.

It is important not to confuse epileptic seizures with the very common 'febrile convulsions' which are usually the result of a sharp rise in a child's temperature, caused by a severe cold or perhaps teething. Most children grow out of these. Some children also have a habit of holding their breath when they are shocked, angry or frustrated, to the point where they actually pass out. Again, this is not serious or harmful and most children grow out of it.

## Sharing care

Whether you are working outside the home or not, you may need or want to share the care of your child with others. This can be done on an informal basis, with grandparents, friends or neighbours taking over for a time, or you might want to work with a childminder. A survey in 2005 by the National Childminding Association found that almost a third of registered childminders were caring for a special needs child or children. Some undertake special training – for example learning a sign language like Makaton. Others are able, with training, to offer full-time childminding or part-time care even to children with the most complex needs, including those who have to be tube-fed.

Childcare can be arranged informally, by asking people you know. Or your local council can give you information on childminders in your area who have places available.

'Under the 2005 Disability Discrimination Act, childminders must make reasonable adjustments to accommodate children with disabilities,' says a spokeswoman for the National Childminding Association.

Childminders offer one-to-one care and continuity of care, which is important for children with special needs. Most of the childminders who care for disabled children are part of a 'Children Come First' network. They may work with the local primary care trust or social services and receive specialist support and help, including being visited by a co-ordinator every six to eight weeks. We would recommend that parents look for a childminder who is part of one of these networks.

If a child is very severely disabled, employing a childminder for a few hours or a day a week can give parents the chance to spend more time with their other children, or simply have some time to themselves.

## Getting around

Children with cerebral palsy need to be able to explore the world and take an interest in what's going on around them just as much as children with no disabilities. Attitudes have changed fundamentally over the last few years and the days when no provision was made for wheelchair users or anyone else whose needs were 'different' are behind us. However, getting around with a child with cerebral palsy is not always easy.

A wide range of pushchairs, wheelchairs, indoor and outdoor walking frames and other mobility aids is available and it can sometimes be hard to decide what is most appropriate for your child. Choosing the right product should be a joint effort between you and the professional therapists. Well-known names like Maclaren and Britax produce 'special needs' products like car seats and strollers for children who may need more support and help with positioning. There is also lots of equipment to help children with cerebral palsy develop their mobility. This can come in the form of balls, wedges, rolls and machines resembling adult gym equipment. Taking a look at the relevant websites, for instance <www .newlifecharity.co.uk> or <www.handyhealthcare.co.uk>, will give you an idea of how much help there is out there, though much of it comes at a price!

The NHS Wheelchair Service is there to help you and will maintain and change your child's wheelchair as he grows older or his needs change. You may have to wait for an appointment – ask your physio or OT for a referral – but once you have your appointment, make sure you ask the adviser about all the available types. Parents recommend doing some research on the Net or contacting sources of independent advice such as the Disabled Living Foundation (contact details on p. 99) rather than simply accepting what is offered.

There is also a charity called Whizz-Kidz (contact details on p. 102). They can provide a range of powered, manual and recreational equipment which can be customized for individual needs. They can also provide tricycles and bicycles and offer wheelchair training and advice for parents, whether you are getting equipment from them or buying it privately. Whizz-Kidz has mobility centres in the West Midlands, the North East and east London. They recommend that you try the NHS service first and apply to them if the product you want is not available.

Car seats specially made for children who need extra support are also available from mobility equipment suppliers.

Some parents find that their children react badly to being placed into a new kind of seat, whether it's a pushchair or a car seat. Children with spastic cp may stiffen and suffer from painful muscle spasms, and those with athetoid cp sometimes find it hard to adjust to new types of seating. If your child finds sitting uncomfortable, painful or distressing, the result can be tears, screams and distress all round, not least for you. If your child refuses to travel in his or her buggy or car seat, ask the advice of health professionals. You may be able to work out between you just what the problem is. Tips from parents, aimed at relaxing children before any trip, range from a little gentle stretching before placing him or her in the seat to the use of a favourite CD in the car player. Cranial osteopathy, as mentioned in the last chapter, can be helpful in relaxing a tense, troubled child. Travel-sickness might be part of the problem. If your child associates being in the car seat with nausea and sickness, one of the many over-the-counter child-safe medications available may help.

Around 8,000 wheelchair-adapted cars are sold in the UK every year. While your child is still small enough to be lifted into a car seat, you may be able to manage perfectly well with an ordinary family car. Depending on the degree of disability, an 'adapted' vehicle may need added cushions, supports or special seat belts, up to and including 'transfer equipment' as your child gets older and needs to be moved from his or her wheelchair into the car. SCOPE can offer advice on this, as can websites for people with disabilities such as <www.youreable.com>.

The Motability scheme (contact details on p. 100) is a long-established, non-profit-making organization which enables people with disabilities to lease or buy a car. It is possible to apply on behalf of a child aged three or older who is entitled to the higher-rate mobility component of Disability Living Allowance (see p. 99). According to Motability, most of their customers choose their contract hire scheme which enables them to choose a new car every three years. See their website for details of how this works.

A car which is used *only* for transporting someone with a disability is exempt from road tax, but if the driver or 'nominee' uses it for his or her own purposes too, road tax must be paid. Call the DVLA helpline or check the Directgov website (contact details on p. 102) for more information about this. As far as parking is concerned, Blue Badge schemes vary around the country. Generally Blue Badges, which enable drivers to park in places where parking is normally restricted, are available to those who are entitled to the higher rate of DLA, or those who need to carry bulky medical equipment for a child under two. It is worthwhile contacting your local social services department (social work department in Scotland) for more information about this.

Public transport is covered, like all services, by the various Disability Discrimination Acts, but provision varies around the country. Dial-a-ride services, hospital transport and local community transport run by volunteers are also available in most parts of the country. Ask your local council about these. Councils, tourist boards and other attractions can also provide information about accessibility, though you may need to make it clear exactly what 'accessibility' means to you by asking whether there are any steps, and so on. Taking your child on an outing can be frustrating if you find when you get to your destination that you can't get in, or can't see everything you have come to see! (See Chapter 7 for more information about travel and holidays.)

# 4

# Early years education

What happens when your child begins to join the outside world, and needs to attend a pre-school playgroup or nursery school? We have already seen that cerebral palsy affects children in different ways. Some have physical difficulties leading to limited mobility and may be wheelchair users. Other may be only mildly affected. Some may have problems eating solid food or be later than non-disabled children to be toilet-trained. Some may be on medication for epilepsy or another cp-related condition.

However your child is affected, she is entitled to have her educational needs met, just like any other child, and that includes early years education just as it does full-time schooling from the age of five.

The Disability Discrimination Acts 1995 and 2005 apply as much to pre-school settings as they do to schools and workplaces. Early years settings should not discriminate against children with disabilities – in other words, should not treat them less favourably than other children. However, less favourable treatment can sometimes be justified if a nursery has particular entry criteria. For example, a nursery for autistic children might not accept a child with cerebral palsy. Other exceptions might be if accepting a child would involve unreasonable expense, or if the nursery 'could not reasonably know' about a child's disability. You can see that these definitions are open to interpretation, and it is sometimes possible to appeal if you think your child is a victim of unfair discrimination. For example, a nursery may make being toilet-trained a condition of acceptance and this might be difficult for a child with cerebral palsy. SCOPE and parents' forums are good sources of advice on this kind of situation.

A useful first step is for you to get hold of a copy of the government's helpful booklet, *Special Educational Needs (SEN) – A Guide for Parents and Carers*, available from the Department for Children,

Schools and Families (DCSF; contact details on p. 99). This makes the point that 'education' begins as soon as your child goes to nursery or another 'early years setting', such as a playgroup. The most recent law dealing with special needs education is the 1996 Education Act, which established a Special Educational Needs Code of Practice. This must be taken into account by playgroups, nurseries, education authorities and health and social services departments.

The booklet also explains that most children's needs can be met within ordinary nurseries or playgroups (or schools as they get older), sometimes with the help of outside specialists. If this is not the case, the local education authority (LEA) has to make an assessment of your child and may then decide to issue a detailed statement, which describes all the child's needs and the special help which can be provided.

This process can seem long-winded and bureaucratic, but your wishes, as parents, are supposed to be taken into account throughout. Most areas have a Parent Partnership Service which offers local support. Details are listed in the DCSF booklet.

The legal rules about assessments only apply to children over two years old. Assessments and statements are rarely produced for very young children, but once your child is two, either you or the child's nursery can apply in the same way as you can for an older child.

Parents sometimes say that obtaining an assessment, or a statement, can be a struggle but is worth it in the end.

'The person who shouts the loudest tends to get what they need. Or at least, some of it!' was one parent's way of expressing it.

## The Portage system

The National Portage Association (contact details on p. 100) is a home-visiting educational service for young children with special needs, from babyhood right up to school age, and their families. There are around 140 local services in this country. Portage workers, who may be teachers, health visitors, community nurses, social workers, parents or other volunteers, undergo special training and visit families once a week. Their goal is to develop play, communication and relationships and enable children with special needs to take part in everyday life, building on what the individual child is able to do.

## Inclusion

Among local authorities, educationalists and therapists, the buzzword for several years now has been 'inclusion'. It was once felt that children with any kind of disability were better catered for in 'special schools', out of the mainstream, but that is no longer thought to be the case. Organizations such as SCOPE and the campaigning group Parents for Inclusion (contact details on p. 101) have been lobbying for some time for children with cp – and other disabilities – to be fully integrated alongside their peers in mainstream schooling. Local education authorities, in partnership with health, social services and the voluntary sector, now have a remit to make sure that children with special needs are included in ordinary early years provision, including playgroups and nurseries. Every local authority should have an inclusion team or an area special educational needs co-ordinator (SENCO) whose job it is to make sure that all the local providers of early years education are working to include children with special needs.

Jo Cameron, of Parents for Inclusion, says that most of the group's members are parents whose children have gone through mainstream schools. 'We work closely with disabled people and have gleaned from them our approach to both the "medical" and "social" models of disability. We are committed to the social model,' she says.

> The medical model says that disabled people have an impairment and that the solution is to fix the impairment. If that can't be done, that's it. The social model says that it's the barriers in society that disable people, not their impairment.
>
> We believe that these barriers can be crossed and that some children do very well in mainstream nurseries and schools, as long as they have excellent support and a robust statement of their individual needs. Parents who have fought for their children's inclusion feel that they have a better life than those who are over-protected. They become part of their local community,

meet and make friends, get invited to birthday parties and so on, rather than being bussed to a special needs nursery outside the area.

We work in 15 Children's Centres across the country, helping both parents and children. The parents of very young children with cerebral palsy may find that they are living in a specialist atmosphere, in between hospitals and therapists, with very little time for ordinary One o'Clock Clubs. What they need is to become part of an ordinary, everyday group of ordinary, everyday families.

Our parents realize that inclusion is about equality and about the right of every child to belong to his or her community.

## Why is 'inclusion' so important?

SCOPE feels that for children with cp, being included is part of being respected and valued. For young children, it says that inclusion is about fitting the setting (playgroup or nursery) to meet the child's needs, rather than expecting him or her to fit in with inappropriate rules. When you are choosing a nursery or playgroup for your child you will want to find out about the setting's knowledge, skills and experience of disability. Even if – as is likely – they have worked with children with special needs in the past, you are the expert when it comes to your child. Most playgroup leaders and nursery staff are flexible enough to offer appropriate help.

SCOPE and the organization HemiHelp have produced guidelines for early years educational settings. It's worth looking at their websites (details on p. 101 and p. 102) for these if you are looking for a nursery or playgroup for your child, as they give an idea of what is desirable. They say that nurseries should have a positive attitude to disabled children, where the staff support and encourage all children to reach their potential. They say that staff should

- understand the needs of children with cerebral palsy, in terms of the condition and how it might affect a child's learning and development;
- ensure the environment and accessories are accessible for children with cp;
- know where to go for further information and advice;

- have a proactive, planned approach to inclusion generally, rather than reacting to individual referrals;
- take into account the needs of disabled children when making changes to the environment, or buying furniture or equipment;
- review their policies and practices to ensure they don't discriminate against children with disabilities;
- recognize that not all children with cp need one-to-one support;
- treat each child as an individual rather than a batch of needs.

A warm, welcoming atmosphere and a willingness to listen to you when you let them know just what your child can and can't manage to do are really important. Cerebral palsy is such an individual condition that general guidelines are not always appropriate.

There are special initiatives which nurseries can employ for children whose progress seems extra slow or who have particularly complex needs. These are called Early Years Action and Early Years Action Plus, and you can discuss them with the local SENCO as well as the nursery staff.

Nicola Gibson is the Inclusion Manager for the Pre-School Learning Alliance (contact details on p. 101). She is also a former SENCO herself and feels that although inclusion can work very well for most children with cerebral palsy, some – notably those with very complex needs – might be better off in a quieter setting with more experienced and knowledgeable staff.

'I used to be 100 per cent in favour of integration, but if the right resources are not in place it doesn't always work,' she comments.

I worked in an 'opportunity group' for children with hemiplegia. Their parents all wanted them to be integrated with non-disabled children. We worked as a team with the physio- and occupational therapists who came along to advise us on handling and positioning the children, and they did very well. However, I have heard of children with, for example, athetoid cp being put on beanbags for the day, or children being knocked over and perhaps frightened by the boisterous behaviour of the other children, and obviously this is not what disabled children need.

There are fewer special needs playgroups and nurseries than there used to be, and for parents to go to a pre-school and put their child into the hands of someone who has no knowledge of, or experience of, cerebral palsy could be a disaster.

If your child is going to playgroup or nursery it's important to plan ahead. Communication is vital. Talk to the staff and also to your child's key worker, physio, OT and anyone else involved, so that a plan can be made which meets your child's individual needs. If those needs are highly complex – for instance, if you feel your child needs one-to-one care or gastric feeding – it might be best if he or she is the only child in the group who does. Inclusion can benefit children with cp. They enjoy the interaction with other children and the happy atmosphere, as long as they get the support they need.

I feel that parents should have the choice between inclusive and special needs playgroups but they often don't. It depends what is available locally.

Children of this age are not generally unkind if there's someone with special needs in the group. They might ask questions, such as 'Why can't Sam stand up like I can?' but that is just curiosity. It is best not to make a huge issue of it but simply to answer, honestly, that Sam's legs don't work very well and that he uses a standing frame when he stands up. Small children will then simply accept Sam's disability.

Chris Johns runs Lewisham Opportunity Group in south London, an inclusive pre-school which was founded in 1981 and looks after 20 children at each session, half of whom have disabilities ranging from Down's syndrome to severe cp.

'The group was started because of two very young mums who had disabled children and wanted them to be treated as normally as possible,' says Chris.

The group works because we are highly staffed. There are never fewer than seven staff on duty and usually eight or nine, some of whom have worked here for a long time. We also have a purpose-built building which is totally accessible. We are Makaton-trained and use signing with all our children, plus a lot of symbols, and we have a 'soft room' for physio.

Inclusion works very well if each individual child has the support they need, and that comes down to resources. A child with severe cp who has to have help getting around will need a helper if he is to be included in all the activities. Without a high staff-to-child ratio, it just wouldn't work. It isn't enough to say that children with cp are welcomed to nursery or playgroup, they also need to be encouraged – and enabled – to take part in everything that's going on.

Our children are very accepting. Little ones often don't notice any differences, and if they do, we explain in very simple terms. They can be very protective and caring too.

What advice would Chris give to parents looking for pre-school settings for a child with cerebral palsy?

'Do your homework!' she says.

Look at the needs of your child first. The staff need to be knowledgeable about his condition, and ideally have some training. Some playgroups, unfortunately, don't accept children who are not toilet-trained, though obviously we do.

I do home visits before children come to us, which helps both us and the parents. Coming to a group like ours may be a first real step into the outside world. I'll talk to everyone else involved with the child's care – the physiotherapist, perhaps a Portage worker, and also see what equipment the child has at home. A group like ours can provide a support network for parents as well, as they realize they are not alone.

## How parents may feel

Not every parent is as enthusiastic about inclusion as the professionals. 'It's good for some children, but not for my child!' is a fairly typical comment. Among the parents I spoke to for this book, experiences and reactions were very mixed.

'Our local authority runs two nursery–primary schools for children with special needs,' says Rosemary.

One is specifically for children with learning difficulties and the other for those like Gemma whose needs are more physical. She wouldn't be able to cope with mainstream school. She can't speak and she can be very disruptive, shouting and laughing uncontrollably and inappropriately. She started her special needs nursery at three and has been very happy there. A friend's child, who is less severely affected by cp, is in mainstream school but it just wouldn't work for Gemma.

'Molly attends the local mainstream nursery and they have been fantastic,' says Chris.

> Molly has no controlled body movements and can't yet sit up, but she enjoys being with the other children and the staff include her in everything. However, our local authority have done their best to make things difficult by making the nursery jump through various health and safety risk assessments.

'Iain has no mobility at all and can only use his left hand. He attended mainstream playgroups and then a special needs nursery. Both were okay – I don't have strong feelings about inclusion either way, to be honest,' says Jacqui.

There is clearly a demand among some parents for specialized playgroups and nursery schools and they do exist. To find out if there is provision in your area, you could get in touch with the Family Information Service of your local council, or one of the parents' support groups such as Contact a Family (contact details on p. 99).

First Step is an opportunity group in east London for local babies and pre-school children with special needs, including cerebral palsy. It was opened in 1988 in response to requests from parents who felt that both they and their children would benefit from a group for families in similar situations, and where their child would not be the odd one out. Their spokeswoman Jill Webb comments that twenty years ago, the word 'inclusion' was simply not used.

> Our group was set up because parents of children with disabilities felt isolated. These days, playgroups and nursery schools can't refuse to take children with special needs, but it should be the parents' choice. Inclusion can work well as long as the funding and expertise is there, but we offer the specialized support that some parents and their children need.
>
> We run family sessions, helping parents to come to terms with their child's disability, and we always put the child first. Children with cerebral palsy pass all the same milestones as other children and a group like ours can empower them, gradually, to face the outside world. We offer a sanctuary where no-one stares or comments, and no-one bats an eyelid if a three- or four-year-old is still in nappies at night.
>
> We welcome pre-school-age siblings with or without disabilities

and we also run 'sib clubs' for the eight- to 13-year-olds, who can often feel very left out or be embarrassed or resentful of brothers and sisters with special needs. Although, of course, they can also be very protective.

Helping children to mix with others and learn what is or isn't acceptable behaviour is part of early years learning, and First Step staff are able to tackle behaviour issues like tantrums, screaming, spitting and general 'naughtiness'.

'Babies with cp often do cry a lot, especially if they have painful muscle spasms,' Jill says. 'We run a specific group for children with behaviour problems, where we try to show them what is and isn't acceptable, usually by positive reinforcement techniques and lots of praise when they get things right. We try not to be negative.'

Senior staff at First Step are trained in the use of medication for children who may need it. When a child joins the group an individual healthcare plan will be drawn up, often with the help of the family's health visitor, and all medication is kept in a locked cupboard. As with all pre-school settings, there is a high staff-to-child ratio – six or seven staff to every ten children – which means that everyone gets plenty of individual attention.

'Early intervention is important for children with disabilities,' Jill comments. 'We are able to deal with some very complex medical conditions here. Some of our children are enabled to go on to mainstream school but I think there is definitely a place for dedicated special needs provision.'

# 5

# The school-age child

All children, including those with cerebral palsy, are entitled to an appropriate education which meets their individual needs. It is now unlawful for schools to discriminate against disabled children and, according to the Department for Children, Schools and Families' booklet *Special Educational Needs (SEN) – A Guide for Parents and Carers*, the basic principles are that:

- all children with special educational needs should have those needs met;
- the special educational needs of children are normally met in mainstream (ordinary) schools;
- your views as parents should be taken into account and the wishes of your child should be listened to;
- you have a vital role in supporting your child's education;
- children with special educational needs should get a broad, well-balanced and relevant education, including the National Curriculum for children aged five to 16.

The days when children with any kind of disability were shunted away, out of sight, and not expected to mix with their peers or play any part in ordinary community life are, thankfully, long gone. Many children with cerebral palsy, like other children with special needs, are well integrated and happy in mainstream schools, and do well there. But because cp is such an individual condition, there will probably always be some children who do better in 'special schools' with specialist staff. Most special schools have a very high staff-to-pupil ratio so that the children get a tremendous amount of individual attention. With the best will in the world, it can be hard for a teacher working with 30 children in a class, or one who has not had extensive training in special needs work, to give a child with complex needs the same kind of appropriate one-to-one support.

It's difficult enough for the parents of non-disabled children to be sure the school their child attends is absolutely the right place for him or her. It's much more complicated when your child has physical impairments or learning or behavioural difficulties as well.

## Assessments and statements

Your child may well have had his 'special educational needs' identified before he is old enough for full-time school. For example, this could have happened when he was at nursery, or in another early years setting. If he hasn't, this will happen when he goes to school. Generally, the earlier a child's needs are identified the better, as the necessary help – whether this means easier access to the school buildings, special equipment or a one-to-one helper – can then be provided.

Just as in early years settings, particular initiatives can be put in place for children with special needs. These are called School Action and School Action Plus and will normally involve your child's class teacher with you, the parents and/or carers, and the local SENCO or special educational needs co-ordinator, working out just what would help your child most. External help, for example an educational psychologist, may sometimes be brought in.

The next step comes when the school asks the local education authority to carry out what is known as a 'statutory assessment'. This is a more detailed investigation aimed at finding out exactly what your child's needs are and how they can best be met. As parents, you are entitled to ask for an assessment even if the school does not do so. The LEA is supposed to tell you within six weeks if they are prepared to do this and should give you the name of a person at the LEA (your 'Named Officer') who is your contact there.

If the LEA decides your child needs an assessment, it should take no longer than six months. Once it has happened the LEA can *then* decide whether to issue a 'statement'. The full name for this is a 'statement of special educational needs'. It is a complex, six-part document setting out in detail what your child's needs are and how they will best be met, including which school your child will attend.

The whole process can seem long-winded, bureaucratic and, of course, stressful for both you and your child, but most parents who have obtained a statement say that it's worth it in the end! You have the right to appeal against the authority's decision at all stages, up to and including suggesting a different school for your child if you feel that it would be more suitable (see Toni and Josh's story on p. 48).

The DCSF booklet gives lots of information about how the statementing process should work. It also lists the contact details for Parent Partnership Services in every area. The campaigning and support group Contact a Family (contact details on p. 99) also publishes booklets, *Special Educational Needs – England* and *Special Educational Needs – Wales*, which can be read alongside the official one to give a really clear picture of parents' rights at this point. SCOPE (contact details on p. 101) can also help parents with questions about education for children with cerebral palsy.

## Choosing the right school

Perhaps you feel that attending the local primary school, with some extra help, would be best for your child. On the other hand, it could be that your child has more complex needs which you believe would be better catered for in a special school. In either case you need to visit the school, meet the head and staff, ask questions, and get a 'feel' for the place where your child will be spending his or her time. It is also a good idea to talk to your local SENCO to find out about the provision for, and attitudes to, special needs children in local mainstream schools. There may be one or more schools in the area where children with cerebral palsy are particularly welcomed and well catered for.

One useful website, <www.ukfamily.co.uk>, has come up with a list of the kind of questions you might ask a SENCO or the head teacher. These could include:

- What is the attitude of staff and pupils to including children with special needs?
- Is any special provision made for such children around the school?

- Have staff attended any recent training courses to work with special needs children?
- Do any teachers have specific qualifications for working with special needs children?
- How do the staff ensure that special needs children are included in all activities, trips and so on?
- How are the children's successes recognized?
- Is there any special pastoral care for disabled children?
- Are there other children in the school with cerebral palsy or similar impairments?
- Will my child be excluded from any activities?
- Are there classroom assistants or special equipment?
- Can teaching methods be adapted to suit my child?
- How does the school deal with behaviour management and discipline issues?
- Is there anywhere quiet for a child to calm down if necessary?
- Can the staff administer any medication my child might need?

Above all, you will need to feel that the staff, the SENCO and the other children are warm and welcoming and positively *want* your child to be part of their school.

## Advantages of inclusion

The Alliance for Inclusive Education (contact details on p. 98) believes that children with special needs should be educated in mainstream schools which are committed to removing all the barriers to full participation. It is not in favour of 'integration' – which happens in some local areas – where children with special needs are accepted as long as they fit into the school's existing structures and environment, and it is opposed to 'segregation', which it defines as sending special needs children to special schools.

Inclusion is standard practice in some countries, like Italy, and also in some states of the USA.

The campaigning group Parents for Inclusion believes strongly that children with special needs, including cerebral palsy, should go to ordinary mainstream schools alongside their peers without disabilities.

'There does have to be excellent support and a robust statement to support the child,' says a spokesperson.

> Parents who have fought for inclusion for their children tend to feel that they have a better life and a better education than those who have been over-protected, even if they don't get as much therapy.
>
> Most of us are the parents of children who have gone through, or are going through, mainstream education. Some schools are not yet ready for children with very complex needs, but parents who are determined that their children should be included have actually managed to change the schools!
>
> If you go to the local school, you meet other, local parents and other, local children and are not cut off from your community. Our children learn to be streetwise like any other children. They make friends locally. There are so many aids to communication now that even children with complex needs can be integrated into mainstream schools.
>
> We run courses, lasting three days, called 'Planning Positive Futures' for parents, enabling them to face their fears, look at solutions and the tools which can enable their children to be included.

## How parents and children may feel

Toni's son Josh is seven, one of twins, and severely disabled. He attended a mainstream nursery where the staff were very supportive, giving him one-to-one attention and providing a special seat for him. At four and a half, he went to a special needs school which took children with a variety of impairments, but he has since moved to his present school which caters only for children with problems similar to his own.

'It's important to remember that all children with special needs have different educational requirements,' Toni says.

> Blind children are not taught in exactly the same way as autistic children or children with Down's syndrome. At Josh's first special school, the staff didn't have experience of every kind of disability and we felt he was being babysat rather than learning.

It took Josh's family about a year to have him awarded a place at the school they felt best met his needs, which was just across the county border under a different local authority.

Everyone agreed that this was the right school for Josh except the local authority. Our particular county has closed all its schools for children with severe disabilities and there were arguments between the social services and the health authority about funding. We did get a statement for Josh but found it wishy-washy – it said things like 'he would benefit from' various kinds of help, which could be said of any child, and that he needed some help 'regularly', which could mean anything from weekly to yearly! What we were interested in was Section Four, which named the school the local authority deemed most suitable.

It was important to us that Josh went to his present school so we took our case to a tribunal. We had help from an organization called IPSEA [contact details on p. 100] and also from the Blind Children's Association, as Josh is registered blind. They said the first school did not meet Josh's needs from a visual point of view. The educational psychologist also backed us, and eventually at the tribunal the Chair came down in our favour. It was an expensive and stressful procedure but worth it in the end.

Josh's current school has only 22 pupils and in his class there are just four children.

'It's brilliant. Even the taxi drivers who take him to school can see the change in him,' says Toni.

It is a partially residential school so Josh stays there from Monday to Friday, which means he doesn't get as tired from travelling. It also gives us some respite and time to spend with Ben, his brother. In the evenings the children do all kinds of structured activities, from swimming in the hydrotherapy pool to cookery lessons, to massage, trips out and bike riding. There are medical staff on hand if there are any medical problems and all the staff are trained and experienced in dealing with children with Josh's sort of disability.

They do little things to help Josh as a matter of course. They know his sight is poor, so before they set off for swimming they will touch his hand on a towel. Before they go for a meal they will touch his hands on a knife and fork. Things like that help him to know what's going on all the time. They have lots of wonderful, imaginative ideas to help Josh learn, which might not happen in an ordinary primary school.

Inclusion would not be practical for Josh but that doesn't mean he is cut off from the rest of the world. He goes to a local mainstream school for music and art lessons and loves being with the other children. He goes to Ben's school sometimes. Ben's teachers told the children about Josh and none of them stared or felt frightened, they just see him as Josh. His own school has an 'open door' policy and holds coffee mornings so that parents can meet each other. We also live in a small community so Josh isn't left out of anything that's going on.

Melanie's severely disabled son Jamie goes to a mainstream infants' school, which she says is wonderful. After what she describes as a 'fight' with the education authority, he will now stay there for an extra year. After that he will go to a special needs school to complete his education.

'The other parents have all told me how fantastic it has been having Jamie at the school,' she says.

He has loads of friends, is really popular, gets asked out to tea and parties and is even sent emails! The other kids push his wheelchair and help to prop his head up if it falls forward.

I am sure he would have a harder time in mainstream schools as he got older, though. He can't speak and I think inclusion has its limits for non-verbal children. A boy with similar problems to Jamie's at a local school wrote a poem about being friendless and about the way people talked over his head. It was heartbreaking. Older children can be cruel to anyone who doesn't fit in, and I'd like Jamie to know there are other children like him.

'As a child I soon realized that I just couldn't do everything the others could,' says David, who is now in his early twenties and always attended mainstream schools.

I've always used crutches except for long distances, when I have a wheelchair. I'm pretty mobile and always was, even though I couldn't play football. Cerebral palsy tends to be a very visible impairment so you do get noticed at school.

I always went to mainstream schools, though my parents made sure they were small schools so that I wouldn't get lost in the crowd. I had a good time and was never bullied or treated badly. I had a 'helper' in class although I never had too many problems with my hands and arms. It was always my legs and my balance which was a problem. The other kids just seemed to accept me.

I wasn't the most popular boy in the class but I did make friends, it wasn't hard. And, cerebral palsy or not, I could always stand up for myself! I think one of the reasons I did so well in mainstream school was because I am one of eight children! My mum was – and is – a real warrior and always made sure I had exactly the same treatment as all the other children. My family were really supportive all through my schooldays.

I've always thought it must be tougher in mainstream school if you have communication problems, as some people with cp do. I'd say I was treated like all the other children by the staff and the other pupils. I was just the one whose legs didn't work too well.

## How SCOPE can help

Campaigning group SCOPE is committed to the fight for good-quality education and support for all children with cerebral palsy, including those with additional needs. The group has regional Inclusion Teams around the country which can help local mainstream schools organize appropriate support for children with cerebral palsy. If you want your child to go to a local mainstream school, they could be the people to approach.

SCOPE can give advice and sometimes hands-on support in the form of speech and language therapy, including the use of Augmentative and Alternative Communication (AAC) systems for children whose cerebral palsy means they have communication difficulties. It can also advise on nursing care and physio- and occupational therapy, as well as giving general guidance on appropriate education.

Inclusion Teams can also help if there are behavioural issues which need to be addressed to enable your child to settle happily into a mainstream school. Children with behaviour problems, sometimes caused by frustration, can often benefit from specialist help, and SCOPE can advise both parents and, crucially, teachers, concerned about behaviour management.

## Tips on behaviour management

Like all children, those with cerebral palsy can become frustrated and difficult when they don't get what they want and can respond to discipline with tantrums, screaming, hitting and biting, self-harming and other challenging behaviours. This sort of behaviour is most common among children who, in addition to cerebral palsy, have learning disabilities or impairments in understanding, so that they find it hard to reason and make sense of their environment.

A child who screams, self-harms, hits out, throws toys, spits or behaves in ways that are unacceptable in class may be trying to communicate or express his feelings of distress, anger, frustration, physical discomfort or pain. A speech and language therapist will be able to teach him alternative and more acceptable ways of making his needs known.

SCOPE recommends that the same behaviour management techniques be used in school and at home, so that the child is treated with consistency and learns what is, and is not, acceptable.

Parents and teachers can learn by observation what upsets their children, even those without speech. It's important to ask yourself:

- What led up to the difficult behaviour?
- What happened during the tantrum?
- What happened afterwards?
- What was the result for the child?

Techniques for managing challenging behaviour in school-age children include 'taking time out' for the child in a quiet environment until he or she has calmed down, teaching particular relaxation techniques, and changing the environment so that the frustrating situation doesn't arise, or the child is simply unable to do whatever it is. For example if he or she throws toys, the toys can be either moved or replaced by soft toys which won't hurt if they hit another child. Working out what the child wants ( a drink? the lavatory?) and providing it is a simple solution. Distraction can also be effective. It's always better to praise rather than blame, rewarding good behaviour rather than punishing bad. It's also important to remember that children with severe cp can tire easily, so some challenging behaviour may be the result of nothing more than tiredness. A shorter school day, or more 'quiet time' in class, might be indicated here.

More detailed information about the causes of challenging behaviour and the best ways of dealing with it can be obtained from the Challenging Behaviour Foundation (contact details on p. 99).

## SCOPE special schools

As well as advising on integrating children with cp into main-stream schools, SCOPE has five special schools of its own around the country. These are generally most appropriate for children with complex additional needs as well as cerebral palsy. Some children attend as day pupils, some as boarders and some as weekly boarders, and short breaks are sometimes possible too. The schools are

- Craig y Parc in Cardiff, which takes children from three to eight years old with very complex learning difficulties;
- Ingfield Manor in West Sussex, which takes children from three to 16 years old and specializes in Conductive Education (see p. 79);
- Meldreth Manor in Cambridgeshire, which takes children between nine and 19 years old with complex needs;
- Rutland House in Nottinghamshire, which takes children between five and 18 years old with a range of physical, sensory and learning disabilities;
- Beech Tree, near Preston in Lancashire, which takes secondary-school-age children from 11 to 18 with special educational needs and severe challenging behaviour.

More information about these schools can be obtained from SCOPE (contact details on p. 101). However severe their pupils' difficulties, these schools also try to make sure that the children are accepted as part of the community.

## Exclusion

In spite of the efforts of campaigners, and the government, whose December 2007 'Children's Plan' expressed a commitment to address the factors holding back disabled children in our education system, it's still a fact that about two-thirds of the children 'excluded' from schools have special needs. The support group Contact a Family says that many special needs children get a raw deal and that children with disabilities, like other children who are seen as 'not fitting in', are more likely to be bullied than their peers.

'Many of our parents feel that there is a lack of training and general disability awareness in schools, and that with better support, exclusion need not happen as often,' says their spokeswoman.

## Bullying

It is only fairly recently that bullying in schools – or outside them, for that matter – has been taken seriously. Previous generations tended to think of bullying as 'just part of growing up' and as something that children should expect, get used to and deal with on their own. Quite apart from the morality of this laissez-faire approach, it is clearly totally unacceptable as well as unrealistic to expect disabled children to 'learn to stand up for themselves'.

Bullying is now, quite rightly, taken a lot more seriously, and most good schools have anti-bullying strategies. Official policy varies in different parts of the UK but it's certainly worth checking with the head of any school your child attends to see what strategies are in place to prevent it. Organizations like Kidscape and Childline (which gets more than 32,000 calls a year from children concerned about bullying) have done considerable research in what it is, why it happens and, most importantly, what can be done about it. A 2007 report from the Children's Commissioner for England reported that disabled children and those with visible medical conditions were about twice as likely to be bullied as their non-disabled peers. In the same year, Mencap reported that nine out of ten children with learning difficulties experienced bullying at some time.

Bullying can be defined as aggressive, hostile or frightening behaviour by a stronger person or a group of people, directed against a weaker or smaller person. Children who are seen as 'different' may be picked on as particular targets, which explains why a child who is a wheelchair user, has a walking frame, wears thick glasses or has poor physical co-ordination may be singled out for unkind treatment.

Bullying isn't always physical, though it can be. Name-calling, cruel teasing, exclusion, tormenting by hiding books or humiliating the child, can also make life miserable. Racist, sexual and homophobic bullying can affect some children. The increased use of technology like mobile phones and the Internet has led to a rise in 'cyber-bullying'. Children are sometimes sent threatening texts or emails, or photos may be taken of bullying incidents and distributed through mobiles or social networking sites.

Bullying matters, because it can scar children for life and leave their self-esteem in tatters. If schools allow bullying to take place they are reinforcing the idea that physical and mental cruelty is acceptable.

If you suspect that your child is being bullied – he may tell you, or you may notice that he seems afraid of going to school – you need to enlist the help of the school staff. Schools should make it clear that bullying of any kind will not be tolerated under any circumstances. Children sometimes choose to bully someone different out of pure ignorance. If that's the case, you might be able to help educate your child's class about cerebral palsy – SCOPE has lots of information which parents and teachers can use. Some schools have a 'buddying' or 'mentoring' system for vulnerable children where classmates learn to help by, for instance, carrying trays in the school canteen or helping with heavy bags. 'Circle time' and Personal Health and Social Education classes can be used to explore 'difference' and teach children about tolerance and understanding.

Your child should also be told that bullying should *always* be reported to a trusted adult and that reporting does not make him a 'grass'!

# 6

# The teenage years

Adolescence is a time of great changes – not just for children, but for parents too! Some of the changes are physical, with 'growth spurts' turning a chubby child into a leggy young woman, or a lad into a deep-voiced stranger who suddenly needs to shave every morning. Others are emotional, with youngsters battling against the authority of their parents and wanting more freedom. And there are practical changes too, realizing that you have another adult, or semi-adult, in the house. It isn't easy for anyone, and having a child with a disability can add further complications.

As we have learned, cerebral palsy varies in its severity, with some young people just having to deal with stiff, uncomfortable limbs that don't work quite as well as they should, and others remaining dependent on their parents and carers for most or all of their physical needs. While the actual brain damage which caused the cp in the first place does not get worse, it can affect young people differently as they grow up, as Liverpool physiotherapist Laura explains.

> As an example, spasticity may not be a problem before a child has learned to walk, or before he goes to school. The impact of increasing height, or weight, on already weak muscles as a child grows can make his cp appear worse. The impact is still greater as the child gets older and heavier, which means that a teenage growth spurt may affect your child's ability to do 'standing transfers' – for example, from a chair to a toilet seat or from one seat to another. This will clearly have an effect on the amount of activity your child can do, and a consultation with his physiotherapist may lead to different types of exercise being prescribed.
>
> Some teens don't want to continue with their physio sessions, and if they have made an informed decision we have to take that on board. On the other hand, if they find their limbs are becoming stiffer and it's more difficult for them to walk, they may come back. Then we can talk about a stretching programme,

gym work or swimming, something that can be integrated into their everyday life. Teenagers are often eager to take responsibility for their own functional difficulties, and it has to be their decision.

Usually, they don't want to be taken out of lessons for physio sessions, or made to feel different from their peers at school. The majority, whatever their difficulties, will go to mainstream schools where they are much more fully integrated than they used to be and where people are much better trained in what physical disability means. Quality of life is not necessarily less for young people with cerebral palsy. A recent European study looked at the services and community facilities in eight different countries and found that the quality of life was the same for disabled and non-disabled youngsters, which is comforting!

So it's important that you, as parents, are prepared for some possible changes in your child's physical condition as he or she approaches the teenage years. You should discuss these with the medical professionals involved in your child's care – and with your child, of course.

## Changing schools

The first big change which affects young people in these years is the move from primary to secondary school. Suddenly, from being in a small local school, perhaps within walking distance of home, where they were always taught by the same teacher in the same class and with the same group of friends, they are pitch-forked into the very different environment of secondary school. They may not attend the same one as their primary-school or local friends. There's a lot more to get used to – perhaps travelling some distance, changing classrooms and teachers for every lesson, taking on new subjects. Add to that the complications which can be involved if you are a wheelchair user, or if you have limited mobility or any other disability, and you'll see that it can be a lot to take on.

It's also worrying for parents. The debates about 'parental choice', and about which secondary school your child goes to, come up every year. Some families, inevitably, feel aggrieved that they haven't been allocated a place in their first-choice school. Some people play the system by suddenly developing a religious faith or even moving house to get into the 'right' school. The whole area becomes a mine-field. Naturally, you want your child to go to a school where he or she is happy and benefits from a good education – so how do you, as the parent of a child with a disability, ensure that that happens?

Much depends on the degree of your child's disability. If she already has a place at a special school, or one of the special needs units attached to a mainstream school, she may be able to continue there for the whole of her school career. SCOPE's schools, which cater for children with the most complex needs, take youngsters right through from three to 18 or 19. If you're looking at your local mainstream schools, what should you look for, in addition to the obvious qualities of good teaching, alert, friendly and caring students and an appropriate physical environment?

Remember that your child's statement of special educational needs should be reviewed annually, and you should discuss the transfer to secondary school with the class teacher and SENCO as well as talking it over with your child. Many young people feel strongly that they want to remain with their friends, or perhaps attend the same school as older brothers and sisters.

Judith describes how her son Robbie, now 15, changed schools.

I went round our three local secondary schools and asked them about children with cerebral palsy, as I wanted to see what would be on offer when Robbie was 11. One school was on two sites and had never had a child with cp. Another had had one once, they thought, but they were a bit vague about it. The third had a girl in Year 11 with cp and they arranged for me to meet her and her one-to-one helper. She told me she was included in everything. We did look at another school, further away, with a very good unit for pupils with physical difficulties, but Robbie was determined to go with his friends.

When he first went, it was after a major multi-level operation so he started with three mornings a week and built up. He was in a wheelchair for the first term, though he now walks independently. He has ten hours of one-to-one help a week, which were used medically at first but are now used academically as he is dyslexic and has problems writing and using a keyboard. I've found it helpful to send round an A4 sheet each year for all his teachers to read, explaining how he is affected by cp. This year he's in the second English and the second Maths group, with one-to-one support. The sports teachers have been fantastic at including him in all sports.

Robbie himself says he is included in everything, and that he doesn't want allowances made for him.

> For the first few months I was in a wheelchair which my friends considered more cool than walking! Everyone wanted to push me. Then I used a K walker which was worse because it was so slow. The school is the one all my friends went to. I took part in two Duke of Edinburgh Awards expeditions last year and they made special allowances when I didn't want them to. They wouldn't let me carry the equipment. I learned to ride a bike last year and I also go swimming, but I don't think I have as much independence as my brother and sister. Mum and Dad are more paranoid about my cycling and stuff.

Rosemary's daughter Gemma is very severely disabled by her cp and has learning difficulties. She didn't have to change schools and, at 17, still attends the special needs unit in the grounds of a local mainstream school.

'There is a link to the mainstream school, but generally it is very separate,' Rosemary says.

> Gemma couldn't cope with mainstream education. She can't answer questions; she uses a headswitch for communication and is very strong-willed, often turning it off if she doesn't want to answer! She is only now beginning to use it for everyday chat and to let us know if something is bothering her. We have had to rely on her facial expressions up until now – one look for 'yes' and another for 'no'. She can be disruptive in a group as she sometimes laughs uncontrollably and inappropriately. She has no independent mobility and uses a wheelchair all the time.
>
> She does love stories and being read to, although it's difficult for us to know how much she understands.

## Bullying

Bullying can be an issue for anyone who is seen as 'different' and, sadly, this can apply as easily to young people with disabilities as it can to those who wear glasses, have red hair, are keener on computers than football or can't afford the latest 'must-have' trainers or mobile phone! Teenagers can be just as cruel as younger children and sometimes more so – more unkind, more violent and with more access to modern technology which allows them to 'cyber-bully'. Some of the anti-bullying tips given in the previous chapter can be adapted by teenagers and, just like primary schools, all secondary schools are supposed to have anti-bullying strategies in place.

Staff should make it clear that bullying of *any* student, for *any* reason, is not going to be tolerated.

Fifteen-year-old Robbie was bullied in Year 8, after he stopped using a wheelchair at school.

'I think this was because although he was still different, he was only a bit different,' says mum Judith.

> He was easy to push over, but most of the bullying was verbal. We spoke to his class teacher and SENCO, who were not a lot of help, but then had a long chat to his head of year, who suggested moving him to a different class where the students were more accepting, and also offered counselling. He didn't like talking to us about it because of the culture of not 'dobbing'.
>
> Now he's in Year 10 the school bullying has stopped but the bus is another story. However, Robbie seems to be able to give as good as he gets.

'They see me as an easy target to show off to their friends. I cope by telling them to f*** off, or ignoring them,' Robbie says. 'I don't want Mum to sort it out because if she tells the teacher that would lose me a lot of respect, and let the bullies know they have got to me.'

Organizations like Kidscape and Young Minds (contact details on pp. 100 and 102) have lots of useful information for both parents and teenagers on coping with bullying.

## Confidence and self-esteem

It isn't easy for any teenager to develop confidence and self-esteem. We can all remember fretting about something – exams, looks, friendships, whether or not we would ever find a boy- or girlfriend, making decisions about the future. Teenagers with a disability may have all those worries, plus additional pressures arising out of their condition. The Royal College of Psychiatrists (RCP) says that children with a long-standing physical illness are twice as likely to suffer from emotional problems or disturbed behaviour as those without. They say that this is particularly true of illnesses which affect the brain, such as cerebral palsy, because

- children with physical disabilities may have fewer opportunities to develop their skills, hobbies and interests;
- they may have missed out on education because of frequent visits to hospital or for treatments;
- they may feel 'different' and hate it.

The RCP's advice for parents is to live as normal a family life as possible and learn to 'let go' rather than restricting your teenager's opportunities. Encourage independence and let your teen mix with others, both disabled and non-disabled. Talk to them about issues like 'peer pressure'. Do they really want to be 'one of the crowd', following one after another like sheep, going 'baaa' when the others go 'baaa'? Teach your teen that it's sometimes worth standing out from the crowd instead, and that it's important to be yourself and do what *you* believe in rather than following the latest fashionable fad! Why not be proud to be different?

SCOPE and other organizations are working hard to make people with disabilities more 'visible' so that they are accepted as ordinary members of the community. Events like the Paralympics provide role models for disabled teens, as do TV programmes like teen soap *Hollyoaks* and Ricky Gervais's *The Office*, both of which have featured wheelchair users among their characters.

## Sex, drugs and the rest

It's only relatively recently that the idea that people with disabilities are entitled to form relationships, fall in love, get married, have children and lead the same lives as the rest of us has been accepted. Even now, the FPA says that young people with physical disabilities can miss out on the sex and relationships education other youngsters get. Either their particular situation is simply forgotten, or it's assumed that the information other teens get is not thought to be relevant to them.

The government's 'Every Disabled Child Matters' initiative calls for all children to receive an education appropriate to their needs, which of course includes appropriate sex education. The FPA (contact details on p. 99) does, of course, have lots of teen-friendly information booklets, many written in the form of cartoons. They tend not to mention disability, although the FPA's current booklet on pregnancy does feature a pregnant woman in a wheelchair on the cover. More appropriate booklets seem to be available for young people with learning difficulties, from both the FPA and Brook, the organization which advises young people on sex and relationships. Brook also has a series called 'Young Disabled People Can . . .' featuring a booklet and posters exploring sex and relationships from the point of view of disabled teenagers (see p. 98).

An organization called Outsiders (contact details on p. 101) runs a 'Sex and Disability' helpline and also a social and friendship club, strictly for over–16s only. Their website has a lot of practical tips and hints for older teenagers, on subjects such as 'Will my drooling put off potential partners?' Outsiders' upfront attitude will not be to the taste of all parents, as discussions include such issues as paid sex for disabled young men.

As always, much will depend on the degree of disability experienced by your teenager. For those only mildly affected, you can discuss tricky issues like relationships, parties, drinking and drugs in just the same way as you do with non-disabled siblings.

'Robbie is the youngest of three so takes his cue about drugs and sex from his older sister and brother,' mum Judith comments. 'We all talk about it but they are convinced they know more than we do.'

Whatever your child's circumstances and abilities, it's important to keep the channels of communication open. Teenagers appreciate being listened to, and having their views respected, rather than being 'talked at' and having parents lay down the law. When it comes to smoking, drinking and drugs, an appeal to their vanity or their budget often works better than dire health warnings. You might remind them that

- snogging a smoker is said to be like licking an ashtray;
- a 20-a-day smoker sees around £1,800 a year going up in smoke;
- drunks are far less safe on the streets at night than people with their wits about them;
- vomiting in the street or wetting yourself doesn't make you look cool;
- there's no quality control on illegal drugs – there's no way you

can know what's in the pills you're buying or what effect they will have;

- people under the influence of drink or drugs tend to make bad decisions about things like driving, getting into illegal minicabs or having sex.

You and your teens can find out more about drugs and alcohol from FRANK, the national drugs helpline (contact details on p. 100).

It's important for even the most severely disabled teen to have a social life and take part in as many ordinary teenage activities as possible. Seventeen-year-old Gemma can't go anywhere independently, but she does go out in a group with other young people with special needs.

'Her school has classes about puberty though we are not sure how much she understands,' says Rosemary, her mum.

> She has a hormone injection to stop her periods, though she still gets emotional once a month. She is doubly incontinent and I take care of her personal hygiene needs, so when she goes out with other people, toileting can be a problem. We take her out to shows and pantomimes, anywhere there is a lively atmosphere, though it can be quite difficult dealing with inappropriate noises she makes, or other people's reactions. She enjoys the cinema and we try to go in quiet periods where other people won't be upset. Outings are easier than they used to be as most places are more accessible, and there are often concessionary tickets for carers.

'The experiences you have as a teenager are bound to be different when you have cp,' says David, who is now in his early twenties.

> I wasn't bullied or treated badly but I didn't go to parties or get drunk when I was 16 as some boys do. I wasn't sure how alcohol would affect me.
>
> I was always pretty mobile and only needed a wheelchair for long distances. My arms and upper body are fine, it's just my legs and balance that can be a problem. Forming relationships can be difficult because physical attraction is the first thing that sparks it off. I have had girlfriends and been pretty amazed they were with me when they could go out with someone physically 'normal'. If I am meant to marry, I'm sure someone will come along!

## Letting go

As a responsible parent, your instinct is always to want to keep your child safe. Young people with disabilities seem – indeed, are – especially vulnerable, so it can seem particularly difficult to let them get out there into the real world and make their own mistakes. With extremely disabled teenagers, this just isn't possible. However, most teens with cp want to be part of ordinary everyday life. The best thing that you can do, as parents, is to teach them to take care of themselves so that they have the skills they need to face whatever challenges come their way.

Young people always push the boundaries and try to grow up, whether that means riding a bicycle or going on a date, before their parents think they're ready. Disabled teens are no different in that respect. The wise parent knows when to let go – as well as when to be there to pick up the pieces if and when things go wrong! Letting go, and teaching responsibility, isn't an event which happens, magically, on your son or daughter's sixteenth birthday. Instead, it's an ongoing process. Confident kids who have always been allowed to make decisions for themselves find it easier to assess risk, avoid danger and ignore peer pressure. Help your child to make the right choices in big things by encouraging him or her to make choices in small things. This builds up self-reliance and confidence, too.

## Thinking about the future

Teenagers, with or without disabilities, should be encouraged to think about their future from the age of 14 or so, or in Year 9 at school. Planning a career can be more problematic for someone with cp, depending on the degree of disability, although recent legislation makes it illegal for employers to discriminate against disabled workers as long as they have the ability to do the job. Universities, too, must not treat disabled students less favourably and must make 'reasonable adjustments' so that they are not at a disadvantage.

Some people find that school and university are more accepting of disability than the 'working world'. Jacqui's son Iain has no mobility at all, although he is able to use a motorized wheelchair and has normal speech. Jacqui says,

I do feel that Iain went through school and college and was then dumped, though he would love a job. He attended a mainstream secondary school with a special needs unit where he got the support he needed. The residential college he attended was not so great and he felt more disabled there than he did in mainstream! The group he was with had a range of learning disabilities too and he felt he didn't fit in.

The government's careers service is now called Connexions; it can give teenagers help and advice about careers and the training required. Schools can often be helpful, organizing careers fairs and work experience for their older students. Further education could be something your teen is considering. Most colleges and universities are very open-minded about offering places to students with disabilities. Connexions employs specialist advisers for young people with disabilities who can give them one-to-one, in-depth support. Your child's school or SENCO should have information about this.

Bear in mind that your teen's statement of special educational needs ceases to have legal standing if he or she stays on at school after the age of 16. However, young people at college are also entitled to extra support if they need it. When your child is 14 and her statement comes up for its annual review, all the educational and health professionals involved, plus the teenager herself and her parents or carers, should be putting together a transition plan through the Connexions service. Connexions can also arrange an assessment even if the teenager does not have a statement. Young people with special needs are also entitled to help from the social services if required, in which case social services should also be involved in preparing any transition plan.

Once your child reaches the age of 16 he or she may choose to

- stay on at school, with the option of doing A levels and then going to university;
- go to sixth-form college or a local further education college;
- begin work-based learning, for example a modern apprenticeship or 'Entry to Employment';
- go to a specialist college for students with a particular disability, or a range of disabilities.

Personal advisers at your local Connexions service will be able to give you and your teenager more information about these options.

# 7
# Making life easier

A great deal of progress has been made over the last few years towards integrating people with disabilities into the rest of society. Much credit is due to organizations like SCOPE for campaigning for the rights of those with cerebral palsy to lead normal lives. New buildings and transport, to give just two examples, now have to be wheelchair accessible. There's a lot of help out there for families who are bringing up a disabled child, but many of the parents I spoke to for this book said there could still be problems finding out what help they are entitled to and accessing the help available.

'I seemed to have to do a lot of jumping up and down and shouting. I could never see why I seemed to have to fight for everything my son needed,' was the way one mum put it.

> Specialized equipment like wheelchairs, standing frames, beds and hoists are all provided, but not always without a lot of chasing up and long waits. The choice is usually non-existent – you get what your county bulk-buys. My son would love a faster, motorized chair and one that is more waterproof than the one he has, but unless we go private, he has no hope of getting it. Constantly asking, begging and more begging can get you down, and waiting for people to call you back who never do can be very frustrating.

The support group Contact a Family estimates that it costs three times as much to raise a disabled child as it does to bring up a child without disabilities. Family incomes are often lower, with only 16 per cent of mothers of disabled children working outside the home as compared with 61 per cent of other mothers. SCOPE agrees that the parents of children with cerebral palsy often have to manage on lower incomes, while their expenses are often higher as there is special equipment to be paid for, often higher heating bills, more expensive childcare, plus the cost of travelling to special schools

Tettenhall Library
Upper Street
Wolverhampton
WV6 8QF
Tel: 01902 556308

Self Service Receipt for Borrowing

Patron: 00415282

Title: Coping when your child has cerebral pals
Item: XB00000000029448
Due Back: 12/11/2018  23:59

Total Borrowing: 1
15/10/2018 16:08:57

Thank you for your custom

or nurseries and hospital appointments. That being the case, it is especially important for the families of disabled children to be sure they are claiming all the benefits they are entitled to.

## Benefits you can claim

As anyone who has ever had anything to do with the benefits system knows, claiming can be fraught with problems. Filling in long, complex forms is enough to daunt anyone, and it's hard to be sure you are claiming the right things and providing the right information. All the organizations campaigning for disabled people are able to offer general advice on benefits. For advice on your specific circumstances, they recommend that you contact your local Neighbourhood Law Centre or Citizens Advice (contact details on p. 99). The government also has a range of advice leaflets on the Department for Work and Pensions website (contact details on p. 99) or you can call the Benefits Enquiry Line on 0800 882 200.

The main benefit you can claim as the parent of a disabled child is Disability Living Allowance, or DLA. This is *non-means-tested* – in other words, you are entitled to it regardless of your family income. It is payable every four weeks and the exact amount you get depends on the level of disability experienced by your child and the amount of help he or she needs.

There are two separate parts to DLA – the 'care component' and the 'mobility component'. The care component is payable if your child needs extra help with personal care because of his or her disability, either physical or mental. There are three different rates, depending on the degree of disability, and the benefit can be paid from the time your child is three months old.

The mobility component is payable to children who have difficulties getting about, as compared with other children of their age.

In order to claim DLA you need an application form, which you can get from your local Benefits Office or the Benefits Enquiry Line (0800 882 200). There is also a DLA helpline on 08457 123456; they can send you a date-stamped copy, and if you return it within six weeks your claim will be considered from the date stamped.

The website <www.special-needs-kids.co.uk> has a lot of useful information about how to fill in the claim form. They make the point that you should let the authorities know exactly what your child's problems are, if possible with backing from some of the professionals involved in his or her care, for example your GP, consultant or physiotherapist. You could even ask a professional to help you fill in the form or ask a friend to help. Don't be afraid to ask other parents for their tips and hints through one of the parents' forums on the Internet. They say that being awarded DLA can be a passport to other allowances and other sources of financial help, so it really is worth making sure you get it right.

There is plenty of space on the form for you to describe your child's difficulties – these could be with eating, sleeping, mobility, bathing, seeing and hearing and making him- or herself understood. Don't underestimate the hard work you and your family and friends put into caring. This is not the time or place to be stoical and insist that you can cope. You and your child are entitled to state help; the authorities are not doing you a favour!

If your claim is refused it is possible to appeal or ask for the decision to be reviewed. Don't give up if you believe you are not receiving the help you need.

Another non-means-tested benefit to which your family may be entitled is a Disabled Facilities Grant, which can be up to as much as £25,000 in England and £30,000 in Wales. This grant is intended to help with the cost of adapting a home to meet the specific needs of a child or young person living there. The grant is administered by your local authority and is usually based on an assessment by an occupational therapist, who takes your child's disability and all the circumstances into account before deciding on what adaptations might be needed. These could include

- providing ramps and widening doors to facilitate wheelchair access throughout your home;
- adapting existing washing, bathing, showering and toilet facilities (for example, providing a ground-floor shower and/or toilet);
- installing a stair lift, electric bed or hoist;
- possibly even building an extension to provide suitable facilities.

If your child needs this kind of help, you should check with your local council how applications are made. Don't start doing any work until you have had the go-ahead from the council. It can take time to get an assessment appointment with an occupational therapist and then even more time before the work is authorized, still less completed, but do persevere. Once you have been approved for a Disabled Facilities Grant, the work has to be completed within one year.

As well as these two important benefits there may be other statutory help you can claim. You may be entitled to Carer's Allowance as the carer for a disabled child or young person. Contact Carers UK (contact details on p. 98) for more information about this. Carer's Allowance is the main benefit for carers, and to qualify you need to fit certain criteria:

- You must be 16 or over.
- You must 'care' for 35 hours a week or more.
- The person you're caring for must be receiving particular benefits, such as DLA.
- There are restrictions on how much you may earn if you are working.
- You must live in the UK and not be a full-time student, or in receipt of certain other benefits.

Depending on your income, you may be entitled to other – means-tested – benefits, for example Income Support, Child Tax Credit, Housing Benefit and Council Tax Benefit. Exactly what you will get will depend, of course, on whether you are working, whether you have savings and whether you have paid the correct level of National Insurance contributions while in work. Again, the Benefits Enquiry Line (0800 882 200), Citizens Advice or your local welfare rights unit will be able to give you advice tailored to your individual circumstances.

Other benefits you may not be aware of include VAT relief on items like wheelchairs or other equipment if it is to be used to benefit a disabled person. Contact HM Revenue and Customs (contact details on p. 100) for more information about this. There is also the Family Fund, financed by the government but administered by the Joseph Rowntree Foundation, which was set up to help families with a disabled child (contact details on p. 99). The Family Fund exists to help families who are on low incomes or in receipt of benefits, and who have severely disabled children, to have choices and opportunities to enjoy everyday life. Grants may be given to pay for things like computers, driving lessons, holidays, travel costs, washing machines – the kind of things which do not come under ordinary statutory provision but which may be difficult for low-income families to afford. In order to apply for a grant your child must be severely disabled and aged up to 18.

## Direct Payments

Parents often say that obtaining state help for children with cerebral palsy is a difficult bureaucratic process and that provision varies depending on where you live – the so-called 'postcode lottery'. It was partly to make this easier and give families more choice that the government introduced the 'Direct Payments' scheme.

The government's booklet *A Parent's Guide to Direct Payments* gives all the details and is available from the Department for Children, Schools and Families helpline (contact details on p. 99). The booklet explains that Direct Payments are a way of arranging social care services for disabled children and young people by giving money to parents or guardians to manage the care them-selves, rather than having the local council planning care services on their behalf.

The advantages are that you and your child may not have to wait so long for the service to be available; sorting it out yourself may result in a more flexible arrangement that suits you better; you may be able to plan something locally rather than having to travel; and you will be in control. However, it also means you, as parent and carer, may have to do more work in arranging care – so it's up to you if you think it will suit your family's circumstances better.

## Charity grants

In addition to the provision of state support for children with dis-abilities, there are charities that may provide extra help. SCOPE can help you to find out about these through its 'Funderfinder' scheme, and it also offers tips on how to apply. For example, Elizabeth Finn Care (contact details on p. 99) is a grant-giving charity dedicated to helping people in poverty, including families struggling with the expense of bringing up a disabled child. They can provide long-term allowances, one-off payments and emergency grants, and can also direct applicants to other sources of assistance.

However, charities will not offer the help that should be provided by statutory bodies like the NHS or social services – though they might offer advice on claiming these – so make sure you are getting all your entitlements there first. If you do decide to apply for help from a charity, do your homework. You'll need to make it clear exactly what you need the money for and how your child or your family will benefit. If, for example, you are applying for a grant for a more sophisticated wheelchair, take a look at several catalogues or websites so that you know which model will be most suitable for your child's needs and where the best offers on price are to be found.

## Private fund-raising

SCOPE also has useful information on raising funds yourself to pay for special treatment and/or equipment. It's hard work and can be a lot more complicated than you might think. It is also extremely time-consuming and you will probably find you need a team of helpers, whatever the fund-raising event you are running. It's extremely important to keep meticulous records of where the money comes from and where it goes – into a separate, dedicated bank account. Regulations about charity fund-raising can be complicated. Any street or house-to-house collection may need permission from your local council or even the police. Running an event such as a summer fete or jumble sale might require health and safety involvement, an entertainment or alcohol licence, injury or accident insurance and a first-aider on hand. Having said all that, fund-raising for a local child can be extremely successful, especially if you manage to involve local press, radio and TV.

## Who provides the equipment your child needs?

Generally, your local health authority and social services department have a legal duty to provide aids and equipment to anyone with a disability, including children. As you would expect, it is normally the health authority which provides equipment to meet nursing and medical needs, and social services who are responsible for providing aids to daily living. Once your child is old enough for school, the school or education authority may also be involved in providing special equipment ranging from adapted seating to 'writing boards' and things like computers.

An assessment of the equipment your child needs is usually made by an occupational therapist, who will be able to advise you about suitable equipment for daily living and for managing better within the home.

In addition to any statutory provision, there are lots of companies and organizations offering, and assessing, aids to make the lives of disabled children and their carers easier. The Disabled Living Foundation (contact details on p. 99) can offer free and impartial advice on all kinds of equipment. Assist UK (contact details on p. 98) runs a countrywide network of Disabled Living Centres where equipment may be tried out. Commercial companies like Hearing and Mobility (contact details on p. 100) have catalogues of equipment ranging from highly expensive electric beds to small but handy gadgets which might be useful in helping older children to achieve independence.

## What parents say

Getting the health professionals who are involved in your child's care on your side is a huge help when it comes to accessing special support and equipment. Other parents can also offer tips and hints which can prove invaluable. Here's what some parents had to say.

> There's a very good unit at our local hospital for disabled children and Gemma was able to try out lots of equipment there. We have had excellent support from our paediatrician, especially when it came to all the red tape and paperwork. I seem to have given exactly the same details of Gemma's needs to so many social workers! But things are definitely

better for disabled youngsters as far as getting out and about is concerned and there are often concessionary tickets for carers too.

Our local hospital has been very good for Darcey. She has a special pushchair and wheelchair and lots of other equipment. Our key worker brings us special toys for her to try and she has just been measured for a walking frame. I have also had driving lessons so that I will be able to drive her to her appointments.

Our local health authority have provided seating, wheelchairs and sleeping boards for Molly. She has four-limb cp, has no controlled body movements and cannot sit up. She attends a local mainstream nursery and they have funded a special seat for the time she is there. We have been raising funds privately to help buy additional equipment for the nursery. My office, Molly's grandma's office, my local rugby club and the radio station have all joined in and been very supportive and enthusiastic.

## Travel and holidays

Now that provision for disabled people on public transport and everywhere from shops and restaurants to hotels, both in this country and abroad, has improved so much, it's disheartening to hear from parents that family outings, or 'getting away from it all' on a family holiday, can still cause problems.

'We do find that family outings are hard work and that what some people label as "wheelchair accessible" is not!' says Jacqui.

Going to the cinema usually means one half of the family sitting at the back and the other half sitting with Iain, as the wheelchair spaces are invariably right at the front. Not many people would choose to sit that close to the screen. Eating out is not always a lot of fun as most places pack in as many tables as they can, which means that Iain's chair effectively blocks the walkway. He also needs to be fed, which can make it difficult for one of us to relax and enjoy our meal.

'We've stopped going on holiday after a few disappointments,' says Rosemary. 'Even places which claim to be wheelchair friendly don't always work for us, and Gemma needs a bed with sides on as she might roll out.'

All our parents emphasize how important it is to check before going anywhere that there is proper access for a wheelchair and that there are accessible toilet facilities if you need them. There are lots of guides for disabled travellers, so doing your homework before you plan a trip is much easier than it once was. There are also companies which specialize in providing holidays for families with a disabled child, and summer-camp type trips for disabled youngsters to attend without their parents. Vitalise, for example (contact details on p. 102) has holiday centres in different parts of the UK, including one near Southampton which can cater for 16- to 17-year-olds, and an activity centre in Cornwall which can take families with children as young as six. Activities such as rock-climbing and canoeing are available, and there are self-catering lodges which are fully accessible.

Break (contact details on p. 98) offers low-cost family holidays for children and adults with learning disabilities in their holiday centre in Norfolk, as well as self-catering chalets in Devon for special needs families. The beach there is wheelchair accessible but no care support is provided. They also have a holiday cottage in Normandy, with a ground-floor, wheelchair-accessible bedroom with a hospital bed and fully accessible toilet facilities.

Tourism for All (contact details on p. 102) has a special section on UK holiday accommodation suitable for families with a disabled child. Their online listings give lots of information on exactly what kind of disability can be accepted, what special facilities can be provided, including wheelchair-accessible accommodation, and helpful details such as staff who can use sign language.

Enable Holidays (contact details on p. 99) is a company which specializes in holidays in both Europe and America and checks out all the accommodation, resorts and travel arrangements to be sure that they really are suitable for disabled travellers. They can put together tailor-made programmes for families with special needs.

Among non-specialist holiday companies, Center Parcs seems to get good marks for its accessible facilities (contact details on p. 98).

Local tourist boards in the UK all have booklets detailing which of their attractions are accessible to wheelchair users. If you are using public transport, the Traveline number and website (details on p. 102) has information about accessibility on bus, train and tram services all round the UK.

If you are planning to travel further afield, the Air Transport Users Council (contact details on p. 98) has advice for anyone travelling by air with a disabled passenger. All UK airports now offer ambulifts, disabled toilets and wheelchair assistance, and most airlines will carry your child's wheelchair, though they may ask you for its dimensions in advance. The main advice they give is that you should let them know in plenty of time if a member of your family has special needs so that he or she can be accommodated. Ideally you should discuss your requirements at the time of booking. Bear in mind, too, that security regulations change from year to year, and you should be certain before you travel that any special food or medication your child needs can be taken on board in hand luggage.

Equipment and adapted cars can often be hired in resorts abroad, and specialist companies for disabled travellers can give you information about this. SCOPE also has details of insurance companies specializing in holiday insurance cover for disabled travellers.

# 8
# Treating cerebral palsy

There is, at present, no 'cure' for cerebral palsy, so anyone who claims to be offering any kind of miracle therapy should be treated with extreme scepticism. SCOPE, for example, says on its website that it does not endorse or recommend *any* of the available treatments or therapies. SCOPE also cautions that if you are planning to take your child for any kind of treatment, you talk it over with medical professionals first. The various parents' forums on the Internet, like <www.specialkidsintheuk.org>, are also good sources of information and opinions about treatments that can be helpful.

You always have to remember that cp is an extremely individual condition. Because no two children with cp are affected to the same extent or in the same way, treatment of any kind should be individually tailored for the child. What helps one may not help another. Having said that, there are therapies and treatments which some parents find beneficial. We looked at some of them in Chapter 2, including cranial osteopathy, which often comes up in parents' forums as helping to soothe and relax tense, crying babies. Massage can also help.

Depending on your child's needs, the healthcare team involved with his or her care should include a physiotherapist, an occupational therapist and possibly a speech and language therapist. It helps to be clear about what these professionals actually do.

## The healthcare team

### Physiotherapists

Physiotherapists are concerned with human movement and with maximizing the potential of every patient. Physios play a central role in the management of children with cerebral palsy, often from birth and certainly from the time of diagnosis. A physiotherapist will assess the child and record his or her development over the months and years, and will then devise a personally tailored treatment plan to teach the child

- how to control his or her head movements;
- how to sit, roll over, crawl and walk if possible;
- how *not* to use abnormal movement patterns.

The physio will also help you by showing you the best way to handle your child at home when you are dressing, bathing and feeding him or her. Physios do work holistically, looking at the whole picture of your child's medical history, present lifestyle and particular needs, and taking them into account. New forms of physiotherapy are being developed all the time, and some physiotherapists have additional qualifications in complementary therapies such as acupuncture, massage or craniosacral therapy.

### Occupational therapists
Occupational therapists (OTs) work with both disabled children and adults and their families, helping them to do things that are important to them. This may involve offering advice on adapting a home to make it more suitable for a wheelchair user and on obtaining equipment to make life easier for children and carers. Or it could involve showing new and more appropriate ways to do things according to the child's abilities.

As an example, an OT might offer advice on a suitable wheelchair and also on widening doorways and creating ramps both at home and at school or nursery. For a child with limited control over hand movements, a special switch might allow him to operate his own chair and an adapted keyboard might help him to take part in school lessons and produce 'written' work on a computer screen rather than on paper. Like the other therapists, OTs often liaise between medical staff, parents and teachers as well as the children themselves.

### Speech and language therapists
Speech and language therapists work with children – and adults – who have communication difficulties. They also help those who find eating, drinking and swallowing difficult because their facial and throat muscles are affected by cp.

Difficulties with chewing and swallowing can be a serious problem for children with cp as they can develop lung infections if food 'goes down the wrong way'. Careful positioning and handling can make mealtimes more comfortable and less stressful for children and their parents, and speech therapists can offer advice on this. (See Chapter 3 for more information about possible solutions for this kind of problem.)

Some children with cp have problems learning to speak and some never master it, but that doesn't mean they can't communicate at all. It may be that they can't control their facial muscles, or there may be associated learning difficulties which mean that they have problems using and understanding language.

Speech is, however, only one way in which humans communicate. Body language, eye movements, pointing, looking and facial expression can all be used to make those around the child aware of what he or she is trying to communicate. Speech therapy may be about learning to control the facial muscles or about learning to use other methods of communication, such as a sign language like Makaton or electronic devices. Speech therapists will be able to give you advice about which of these would be most suitable for your child.

## Medication

In some cases, medication may be prescribed to help painfully stiff and tense muscles to relax. This may be a muscle relaxant like diazepam (Valium), which can relax the muscles enough for additional physiotherapy to be given.

A fairly recent development in medication is an injection of botulinum toxin (Botox), the muscle relaxant more usually associated with face-lifts. Botox has actually been used in medicine for 20 years, and in 2000 two products, Botox TM and Dysport, were licensed for use with children in the UK. It's not a cure for cerebral palsy and children need to be individually assessed by a medical team experienced in its use. It can be particularly helpful for children with spastic cp and can be used to treat the characteristic 'tiptoe walking', when a child is unable to put his or her feet flat on the ground. Botox can also be injected into the calf, thigh, hip or arm and hand muscles, reducing stiffness and making sitting, walking, transferring and moving hands and arms easier and less painful. Painful spasms and tiredness are also relieved. The effects of Botox treatment last about three months and should be combined with exercises devised by your child's physiotherapist.

Another possibility is a treatment called intrathecal baclofen therapy, or IBT. This was approved for use in the USA in 1996, and more recently it has also been licensed by the Medicines Control Agency for use in the UK as well, although few children have been treated with it yet. In a two-hour operation, a very small pump is implanted and connected to the spinal cord. It delivers a computer-controlled dose of a drug called baclofen, a muscle relaxant which works by blocking the nerve signals which cause muscles to stiffen.

## Surgery

Orthopaedic surgery is sometimes appropriate for children with cerebral palsy, especially if they find that movement is very painful. It isn't a cure, and is not used to treat abnormal movements or balance problems. However, muscles and tendons which are too short can be lengthened, and these operations are usually performed on the upper leg muscles when the child is between two and four years old, and on the hamstrings when the child is around seven or eight. Children usually recover quickly and well from this type of surgery.

Another operation, called selective dorsal rhizotomy, is sometimes recommended. In this type of surgery, the nerves in the spine which are causing the child's muscle stiffness are identified and removed. The operation should be followed by between three and nine months of extensive physiotherapy, and there can be post-surgical problems such as pins and needles or bladder and bowel difficulties.

## Conductive Education

Many of the therapies offered for children with cerebral palsy are less invasive than surgery and less likely to produce undesirable side effects than drug treatment. One of the best known of these is Conductive Education, an approach pioneered by a Hungarian doctor called Andras Peto, who practised in Budapest just after the Second World War. It is a holistic form of education and rehabilitation for children (and adults) with movement disorders and can help them to lead more active and independent lives. Although it was originally hailed as a breakthrough in the management of all forms of cerebral palsy, it's now accepted that it doesn't help all children, but some do find it extremely useful.

The Birmingham-based Foundation for Conductive Education began offering children's services in 1988. Originally, their specialists had to travel to Hungary to be trained in the therapy, but a BSc (Hons) in Conductive Education is now available at Wolverhampton University. Twenty-five organizations around the country can now offer Conductive Education to children.

Specially trained teachers, known as 'conductors', help children to learn that some movement and co-ordination can be under their own control and that they can discover and solve problems by themselves. Conductors are trained in neurology, disability, physiology, psychology, rehabilitation and motor learning. They motivate children by breaking down each necessary movement into small, achievable steps, and also help the child to *want* to learn the movements, which are then practised over and over until they become automatic. Babies, for example, learn to control their head and eye movements so that they can bond with their parents more easily. Toddlers learn movements which will help them with everyday tasks like dressing and eating. Older children learn the movements required in learning to walk, or perhaps to grip a pencil in order to write. In other words, Conductive Education can help children to develop ways of controlling the effects of their cerebral palsy. Unlike conventional treatments, it is not about having things done *for* the child, or *to* the child. It's about active learning and giving the child the desire and determination to do things for him- or herself.

Conductors work with children, parents and other professionals, helping parents to understand their child's cerebral palsy and encourage greater independence. Their free 'Parent and Child Service' for babies and children up to three

- introduces basic skills and shows how to achieve them;

- helps the child find ways to use motor skills in play;
- advises on appropriate toys and techniques;
- supports the management of everyday activities;
- provides opportunities to meet other parents;
- helps to prepare children for nursery.

These group sessions last one and a half to two hours, once or twice a week. Special arrangements can be made for parents who have to travel a long way. Because Conductive Education is classed as education rather than therapy, it can be funded by education authorities for children over three who have a statement of special educational needs. Families turned down for funding can be helped by trusts and bursaries, and part-time attendance is also possible, so no-one should be put off by lack of resources.

Help is also available for primary-school-age children as well as older children and teenagers. The Foundation reports that some of its original patients, who attended the Peto Institute in Hungary in the 1980s, still come back for sessions now that they are young adults!

Jenny describes her three-year-old son Nathan's Conductive Education sessions as

> like a light coming on. After two appointments, I could see the change in him. He had had physiotherapy before, but the holistic approach of the Foundation made all the difference. He started to sit up, attempted to crawl and use his right hand, and even made noises which he had never done before. Now he talks well. His speech is a bit slurred but I can understand him. He can walk, too, and even tries to run.
>
> The sessions last between one and two hours, once a week, and are very intense. There are lots of activities: looking in mirrors, talking to him, pointing to his features, moving his limbs, shaking and moving different toys, pulling himself along a bench, sitting and standing in particular ways to strengthen his core muscles.
>
> Initially he wasn't sure about it, but he gets so much praise and a sense of achievement and has formed a close bond with his conductors. Nathan has right-side hemiplegia, but there are other children I have seen who are much more seriously affected by their cp. Some of them couldn't sit or stand, and then months later I see them walking with a frame. It has been a very positive experience for us.

## The Bobath approach

The Bobath approach, pioneered by Dr Karel and Mrs Berta Bobath as long ago as the 1940s, is available at three centres in London, Scotland and Wales and also by Bobath-trained therapists who work privately. Its main aim is to encourage and to increase a child's ability to move and function as normally as possible, by helping children to change abnormal movements and postures.

Bobath therapists are all fully qualified as either physiotherapists, occupational therapists or speech and language therapists before they undertake Bobath training after two years specializing in paediatric therapy.

Says one therapist:

> It's very much a holistic approach. We see each child as a unique individual and work with them on a one-to-one basis, analysing the way they move and working out a better way for that child. We look at everything they can do, including their motor, sensory and learning abilities, and also consider the long-term outcome of therapy. As cerebral palsy has no cure they may need treatment throughout their lives. Intervention is most effective when children are young, so little ones may come to us for intensive blocks of therapy in addition to their home-based treatments. They may come less often as they get older, depending on individual need. They may come to us during growth spurts, or even as adults.

Children can be referred to one of the Bobath centres by their GP or paediatric consultant if it is felt they would benefit. However, as with many treatments, whether your local NHS will pay for the treatment varies around the country. Sessions can also be self-funded, although a letter of referral is still needed. Children and young people of all ages, from babies to adults, can all attend the centres.

The Bobath approach can benefit both children with spastic cp, who can learn to become less stiff, and those with athetoid cp, who can learn to have some control over their movements and posture. Children with complex disabilities including visual problems or epilepsy can also benefit. All children are encouraged to explore their environment as much as possible and to participate in games and activities so that they learn to think for themselves, make choices and decisions, solve problems and understand the world around them.

Melanie's six-year-old son Jamie, who has severe and complex disabilities, has been having sessions at the Bobath Centre since he was 18 months old. She says:

> We have had to keep appealing for funding from our primary care trust, and I have also raised funds privately so that he can have weekly sessions. They offer so much more than expert physiotherapy. They talk and interact with Jamie – who is non-verbal – as they would with any other child. I now know he has all the equipment he needs, from shoes to a standing frame to a communication package. Nothing is too much trouble and I don't think I could have coped without them.
>
> They are involved with every aspect of Jamie's care. When he first went there he didn't sleep for more than an hour at a time and it was the Bobath staff who called our local social services and pestered them to get help for us. Their approach is holistic, and everything is under one roof so that those caring for Jamie actually *talk* to one another. Our local community physios and OTs don't seem to do that; the people who see Jamie at home don't communicate with the ones he sees at his school. The Bobath staff are happy to talk to, or see, his teachers and teaching assistants so that he gets joined-up care. They have also put me in touch with other parents whose children have similar problems, which has helped all of us.

## The Scotson Technique

The Scotson Technique, which was devised and developed by psychologist Linda Scotson after her own son was diagnosed with a brain injury, can be studied at the Institute of Advanced Neuromotor Rehabilitation in East Grinstead, Sussex. SCOPE says that this therapy focuses on strengthening a child's diaphragm and reproducing many of the stages of respiratory development on which Dr Scotson believes neurological growth depends.

Put simply, this technique helps to strengthen the muscles used in breathing, so that the child takes in more oxygen. As breathing improves, development becomes more normal, whether the child is mildly, moderately or severely affected by cerebral palsy.

'All children need a responsive, strong respiratory system,' says Dr Scotson.

Every step of our work is well-evidenced scientifically, and pae-diatricians are beginning to support us. We have centres in South Africa, the Philippines and Slovakia, where the neurologists are also very supportive. We work with parents and teach them the tiny, precise movements of the ribcage which result in gentle but effective pressure on the child's lungs. The technique is easy to learn and pleasant for both parents and children. It is a gentle, non-invasive therapy.

Marina's eight-year-old daughter Chloe, who has left-sided hemi-plegia which also affects her right leg, has been attending the Institute for five years. Marina says she can really see the difference this treatment has made.

Doctors and physiotherapists told me there is no cure for cerebral palsy, but I wanted to see some improvement and a good quality of life for Chloe, which was what Linda offered. When we first went there, Chloe's ribcage protruded, her diaphragm was very small, her breathing was shallow and she could only walk a few steps. Now she is in mainstream school, and apart from her walking you wouldn't know she had cp.

Some days are better than others, but when I look at photos of Chloe as she was I can see the progress she has made. The Scotson Technique has made a fantastic difference. We spend about 45 minutes a night on it; Chloe is comfortable watching TV and she hardly feels it. The thera-pists demonstrated on me, so I knew how gentle the movements were. At first I was sceptical because I couldn't see how such slight pressure could make so much difference, but Chloe's body shape has improved so much.

## Other therapies

### Hyperbaric oxygen therapy

The importance of oxygen in the management of cerebral palsy is also the basis of hyperbaric oxygen therapy, which involves the administration of pure oxygen within a hyperbaric chamber, rather like those used by divers to avoid 'the bends'. However, this has so far proved controversial as a treatment for children, although, like the Scotson Technique, the treatment is offered at the Institute of Advanced Neuromotor Rehabilitation and Marina feels it has helped Chloe, in conjunction with the exercise regime.

'Chloe also has regular physiotherapy which keeps her muscles in use, but doesn't actually improve her condition. But all input is valuable,' she comments.

## Hydrotherapy

Hydrotherapy – or just everyday swimming – can benefit children with movement problems too. Gentle exercises practised in water can be beneficial because the water bears the child's weight and can help him or her to enjoy movement without pain, while the resistance offered by the water can help to strengthen weakened muscles.

## Horse-riding

The gentle movements experienced as a child learns horse-riding can also benefit children with cerebral palsy, both physically and psychologically. The Riding for the Disabled organization (contact details on p. 101) is well established in locations all around the country and offers valuable experience to more than 24,000 disabled children and adults every year.

The organization claims that as well as the enjoyment, challenge, friendship, sense of achievement, independence and confidence offered by horse-riding, it also provides genuine therapeutic benefits. The warmth and three-dimensional movement provided by the horse is transmitted through the young rider's body, gradually helping to make it more relaxed and supple, reducing painful spasms and improving balance, posture and co-ordination. Riding can help children with cerebral palsy discover a whole new freedom in movement.

## Swimming with dolphins

Swimming with dolphins is also sometimes recommended, though there doesn't yet seem to be any scientific evidence for its benefits.

## Splints and suits

What your child wears can make a difference too. Australian occupational therapists have devised a form of support called Lycra Dynamic Splinting, individually designed to fit the whole or a part of a child's body and made of strong Lycra. These can help to improve muscle tone, posture and patterns of movement, and enhance quality of life. The company concerned, Second Skin, has an Edinburgh office (contact details on p. 101) and runs clinics in different parts of the UK for those interested in finding out about these products. Referral from a healthcare professional is not necessary.

Specially designed suits, originally used to combat weightlessness in the Russian space programme, are another suggestion. These suits are among the aids used at the Bedfordshire-based Cerebral Palsy Physiotherapy Centre, which was founded by a mum who spent many years researching possible treatments for her daughter. Patented in 2001, the TheraSuits are worn while performing exercises to improve motor development, strength, balance, flexibility and co-ordination. Treatment programmes at the Centre are all individually worked out to address children's particular therapeutic needs. Contact details for the Centre are on p. 99.

### Other possibilities

Research into possible treatments is, of course, ongoing. Deep Brain Stimulation, in which a kind of pacemaker is inserted into an area of the patient's brain, is already used on adults with Parkinson's disease and has been suggested as a possible treatment for dystonia.

Constraint-induced therapy, or CIT, may possibly be useful for children with hemiplegia. This therapy, which involves the 'good' hand being gently restrained so that the person is encouraged to use the weaker one, is already being used on adults who are recovering from a stroke.

## What parents think

Consultant paediatrician Richard Morton advises parents to beware of untried, unproven therapies and says that he has heard of all kinds of odd 'treatments', varying from injections of cells from lamb brains to six-hour crawling sessions or children hanging upside down!

> Generally, the help available on the NHS is good, it's just that there isn't enough of it. I have heard of physiotherapists with

caseloads of 60 children. Conductive Education is helpful for some children and the Bobath approach is very good for some also. Cranial osteopathy can be soothing but it will not change a child's brain function. Other complementary therapies which promote relaxation can be helpful too. Parents need medical professionals they can trust, who will discuss all the possibilities for their child with them.

This was underlined by parents, whose experience of therapies varied a lot, often depending on where they lived.

Josh had cranial osteopathy as a baby which did help him, and Botox on his hips on the NHS, which worked very well.

Building up trust with Matthew's physiotherapist has helped us so much. She now refers us on where needed and is always a listening ear.

Molly has physiotherapy very rarely as there is a shortage of children's physiotherapists in our area. We have been recommended to go to the Bobath Centre but it would have to be at our own expense.

We have a wonderful NHS physiotherapist and Jessica also wears a special Lycra suit which helps to stabilize her trunk and makes her more comfortable.

Joe has had regular sessions of hydrotherapy and I also take him swimming once a week. I have noticed a big improvement in his mobility and he can also stay in a sitting position much longer.

We started off using the Bobath method of physiotherapy, but then we moved and had no choice except for Conductive Education, which didn't help Iain at all.

# 9

# Carers and families

Nothing can really prepare you for the shock of hearing that your child has a disability. Conservative leader David Cameron memorably described the impact of learning that his eldest son Ivan had profound disabilities as 'like being hit by a train'. You can't know in advance how you will react, how you will feel. The shock can temporarily paralyse you and may then be followed by a mixture of confused emotions. These can include grief, as you mourn for the child you thought you were going to have; self-blame (was there anything I or we could have done to prevent this happening?); uncertainty (what is going to happen to our baby?); worry about the future (how on earth will we cope?) and about others' reactions (how will we tell Mum? Dad? the child's brothers and sisters?).

All these feeling are perfectly normal and natural and part of the grieving process – and the emotional roller-coaster you are on *does* resemble grief. All parents-to-be have dreams and plans and ideas about what life will be like when their longed-for baby arrives. There are lots of adjustments to be made if your baby or growing child needs extra-special care, and you wouldn't be human if you didn't go through all kinds of mixed emotions. You could experience an outpouring of love and protectiveness towards this little person who needs you so much, or sadness and even 'why did this have to happen to us' resentment. You are only human, after all, and it can take time to get used to the new reality.

It's really important to accept and recognize your emotions as absolutely natural and nothing to feel ashamed of. As well as help and support from medical professionals and your friends and family, it can be helpful at this stage to look at some of the parenting forums on the Net and realize that you are not alone. Thousands of other parents have faced the challenges you are facing now. They have survived, their families have thrived – and so can you!

'The impact on a family can be massive, and fear of the unknown is always on your mind,' says Chris, father of two-year-old Molly.

It puts a massive strain on mothers and fathers because both are grieving for the child they have lost, while having to cope with all the issues of the one they have.

It would be easy to sink into a dark hole but you can't. Your child really needs your support. You might feel like giving up sometimes, but you can't. Don't be afraid to share and express your emotions, or ask for help. You can't do everything yourself and there are people out there to help.

'The early days were very black,' agrees Melanie, whose six-year-old son has complex disabilities.

Things get better in some ways, and worse in others. Jamie has awful muscle spasms and is in a lot of pain, and has to take drugs to control them and also to help him sleep. I wouldn't have wanted it to happen – and I do regret that my child has cp – but I don't think like that every day. I am blessed to have this special little person who has totally changed the way I think about the world. What would have helped me most in the first year of Jamie's life would have been to be able to talk to other, perhaps older, parents who had been through the same thing.

In the long term, how much your life changes will depend on how severely your child is affected by cerebral palsy. Coming to terms with uncertainty, the 'wait and see' diagnosis which is often given, can be difficult. Many parents report that doctors are excessively gloomy and give parents the worst-case scenario.

'We were told Matt would never walk or talk. He does both, and very well, too, though he has to use a wheelchair to go any distance,' says one proud mum.

Obviously, it is vital to make sure your child is getting all the help he or she is entitled to, up to and including round-the-clock care if need be. We looked at the help available from paediatricians, GPs, therapists and others in earlier chapters. There is help out there, even though 'you have to learn to shout', as another mother expressed it. Battling through what can sometimes seem like excessive bureaucracy and endless form-filling, dealing with a succession of doctors, nurses, therapists and social workers, can seem depressing and demoralizing, but it's worth it in the end if it helps you reach the care your child needs.

You also have to realize that your child is not the only person who matters here. You, and your partner, if you have one, are now 'carers', and you are important too. The members of your child's wider family, including siblings who share your home, are bound to be affected by the changes and challenges of having a disabled child in the family. Who cares for the carers?

## As a carer . . .

You are one of approximately *six million* men and women in the UK who have caring responsibilities of one sort or another. Some are caring for elderly frail parents, others for disabled adults, and many, like you, have the full-time responsibility of looking after a disabled child. It has been estimated that carers – a word and a concept which only came into common usage a few years ago – actually save the state a massive £87 billion a year – the cost of caring for disabled people.

You have rights as a carer, one of the most important being the right to a 'Carer's Assessment' of your own. This is quite separate from any assessment which is made of your child's special needs. You can ask your local social services for this assessment at any time, and should look at it as an opportunity to tell the authorities what they could do to make the task of caring easier for you. The social worker who carries out this assessment should not assume you are able and/or willing to provide the amount of caring that you already do, and should be told as much as possible about your individual circumstances.

When you ask for an assessment, think carefully about what your needs actually are and what the effect of being a full-time carer has been. For instance:

- Do you go out to work? Do you want a job outside the home?
- Are you able to get enough sleep?
- Is your health affected in any way, either physically or emotion-ally? For instance, do you need help with lifting your child to avoid back problems, or do you often feel it's all too much for you? Stress and depression are common reactions to 'overload' and should be mentioned to the social worker. Don't pretend that everything is fine when it isn't.

- Would special equipment to help with feeding, lifting or toileting make a difference?
- Would you like to be put in touch with other carers in a similar situation?
- How much time off from caring do you get?
- Would you like information about respite care for a few hours a week, in day centres, at weekends or for occasional holidays?
- Would you like information about fostering or residential care?

Apart from the Carer's Assessment, you have other rights as well. We looked at the benefits available for those with caring responsibilities in Chapter 7. If you are able to work outside the home, legislation passed in April 2003 states that you have the right to request flexible working from your employer while your disabled child is under 18. This could include allowing you to work from home, to work term times only, or to make some other suitable arrangement. You should request this in writing from your employer, and he or she has 28 days to meet you to discuss the options, with only a limited right to refuse your request.

As a working parent you are also entitled to build up money for the future in a second state pension. The Pension Service (contact details on p. 101) has a useful free guide, *State Pensions for Carers and Parents*.

If you run into legal problems over work, your rights or anything else connected with your child's disability, free advice is available from the Disability Law Service (contact details on p. 99).

There are several organizations which offer help and support to carers, including anyone caring for a disabled child. Carers UK, the Princess Royal Trust for Carers, and Crossroads Caring for Carers are among the best-known names. Not only do they keep carers' needs in the public eye and run campaigns for a better deal, but they also offer practical everyday help.

The Princess Royal Trust for Carers has 144 Carers' Centres all around the country, as well as 85 services for 'young carers'. They can offer information and advice on everything from state benefits and holiday breaks to emotional support if required – anything, they say, that makes it easier for carers to cope. Crossroads, named for the much-loved Midlands-based soap opera which featured a wheelchair user as a leading character, has 123 member schemes across England and Wales, providing 4.7 million care-hours per year and offering a reliable local service tailored to individual needs. Crossroads runs sister schemes in Scotland and Northern Ireland too. Contact details for these organizations are on pp. 98–101.

## Respite care

However much you love your child, 24/7 caring can be exhausting and demoralizing and can leave you little time either for yourself or for your partner and other children, not to mention your wider family and friends. This is why respite care can be a lifeline. The term 'respite care' can mean anything from a couple of hours' break one afternoon a week to give you, as chief carer, time to go shopping, have your hair done, meet a friend for coffee or the cinema or even just have a well-earned nap, to a short break or holiday.

Always ask your GP or social services about respite care and they will let you know what can be provided. As is often the case, provision varies around the country. Some social services departments offer vouchers for short-term breaks. Respite care should be provided as part of your Carer's Assessment. Remember, too, that if you opt for the Direct Payments system, explained on p. 70, you can use part of the money you receive to pay for a carer to come to your home and look after your child at a time that suits you best. Respite care can be 'domiciliary' – in other words, with a carer coming to your home – or 'residential' – with your child going away to be cared for elsewhere – or there may be a special school, day centre or holiday playscheme which will look after him or her for a certain number of hours per week.

Crossroads Caring for Carers aim to help both the carer and the person cared for. Apply to them and one of their trained staff will come to you to discuss what sort of respite care would be most appropriate and suit you best. Respite care is usually provided in your home, and they also run Young Carers projects and holiday playschemes.

The Shared Care Network (contact details on p. 101) also have information on respite care, including 'befriending schemes' and short breaks, which are apparently the kind of respite care most frequently asked for by parents. The breaks they organize usually involve your child going to a trained volunteer's home for an agreed period, which could be anything from one evening a week to one weekend a month, sometimes longer. This gives you a chance to spend time on your own or with the rest of the family, perhaps doing things you wouldn't otherwise be able to do. It also benefits your disabled child by helping to increase her independence and giving her a chance to meet new people, enjoy new experiences and widen her horizons.

## Brothers and sisters

Having a child with cerebral palsy is bound to have an impact on brothers and sisters. Most are loving and protective and willing to share the caring – but they can also feel 'pushed out' and jealous because so much attention is inevitably focused on the disabled sibling. It's hard for parents to find time for their other children when one may be seriously ill and going backwards and forwards to hospital appointments. Single parents have an especially hard time as it may be difficult to make childcare arrangements at a moment's notice.

Research into the effect on children and families of having a member with a disability is inconclusive, but common sense suggests that

- families with a disabled child are sometimes restricted in their ability to take part in everyday activities, especially outside the home;
- parents do need to direct a great deal of their time and attention to the disabled child, often at the expense of the non-disabled siblings;
- children with disabled siblings may experience worry and stress, although they can also learn a lot about caring, tolerance and understanding.

The needs of 'young carers' are beginning to be recognized and many of the carers' websites have support groups for siblings, as do Carers UK, the Princess Royal Trust for Carers and Crossroads. The website <www.youngcarers.net> has a special section for youngsters who help to look after a disabled sibling. They make the point that these children have a right to their own lives too. Many 'young carers' find themselves

- keeping an eye on their disabled siblings in case they hurt themselves;
- helping to feed, wash or toilet them;
- having to look after themselves a lot because the disabled sibling takes up so much of their parents' time;
- helping to care for stressed parents.

Brothers and sisters may feel resentful or angry – even though they love their sibling – and may also be bullied at school because their family member is 'different'.

'We were lucky that Gemma was our first child,' says mum Rosemary.

> Her younger brother and sister have been very accepting, and so are their friends. Spontaneous outings are not possible for our family, though, everything has to be planned and researched first. We are two separate families really – there are sporty things we can do with the other children and things we can do with Gemma.

'It has been hard for Matt's brother. When you are four or five, seeing your brother's wheelchair can drive you crazy with jealousy. We do as much as we can with our other son when Matt is not around,' says Gabrielle.

'Jessica's brother is six and is only just starting to interact with her. It's sad that he will never have a normal relationship with her,' says Annie. 'Jess seems to have hospital appointments at least four times a week and I'm sure Danny feels left out.'

## Attitudes to disability

Out in the wider world, attitudes to disability are changing. SCOPE and other groups campaigning for equal rights for disabled people have done a lot to change perceptions, and children with disabilities are no longer hidden away as if their condition was something to be ashamed of.

There are still some stares and whispers, according to parents spoken to for this book, and occasionally parents' forums report a less than sympathetic attitude on the part of the general public, including bus drivers. Here are some comments

> I wish people wouldn't just stare. They could come up and say hello or ask a question – Josh won't bite! Disabled children are much more visible these days and Josh is young enough to have the cute factor, especially in his funky wheelchair.

> I wish people would ask and show interest rather than just smile and walk away – or worse, ignore us as a family. I am always happy to answer questions about Jess and wish people felt comfortable enough to ask. I see her as my sparky little daughter with the beautiful eyes, not Jess with athetoid cp.

> Some people are great and just accept Iain for who he is. Others treat him like a rather large baby and coo at him. Some just stare. Overall, we have never had any open hostility or bullying. We do get 'oh what a shame and he's so handsome too' but I just smile as they don't mean to be hurtful.

> I'm no different from someone who wears glasses. If someone can't accept that, they're not worth it.

> A friend with a disabled daughter asks the starers if they want a photograph!

> On the whole the general public is lovely – but then, Jamie is an appealing little boy with a cheeky smile. One problem I have found is the battle over disabled parking spaces. I have to use them as Jamie is in a wheelchair, and we have a blue badge, but older people who can't walk very well seem to think they should always have priority, and give us a hard time.

## Looking after yourself

If you are a carer for a disabled child, and especially if you also have other children, a part- or full-time job and a home to run, 'me time' is probably way down on your list of priorities – that's if it ever gets mentioned at all! However, it is very important that carers take time to be good to themselves and take care of their own health and well-being, whatever their circumstances. Running yourself into the ground is not only bad for you, it will not benefit your child either.

Rule 1 has to be: *do not try to do everything yourself.* You are not Superwoman or Superman and there is no ideal for you to live up to. You don't have to be one of the stiff-upper-lip martyrs who insists that he or she can 'manage' when really crying out for help. This book has already shown, I hope, that there are services out there to help you. Use them. If you think your child is getting a poor deal, say so. Perhaps friends could start a campaign for something better. If necessary, involve your local media – papers, radio and TV. Take advantage of every offer of help that comes your way, whether it's from your partner, a friend, your children's granny or aunt, granddad, teacher or babysitter.

Take special care of your own health. This isn't selfish, it's common sense. Most of us nowadays know the rules for healthy eating, even if we aren't always very good at sticking to them. A balanced diet, with at least five portions of fruit and veg a day and fresh, wholesome food, will keep both you and the family fit and full of energy. Keep takeaways, sweets and cakes for occasional treats. It really doesn't take that much longer to prepare a simple meal – filled baked potatoes with salad, for example – than it does to microwave a ready-meal full of fats and additives.

The other half of the fitness equation is, of course, exercise, and that should be part of your everyday routine as well. Make a point of walking to the shops or even to your child's medical appointments if you can. At weekends, go for family walks in the park or a swim at your local leisure centre so that exercise is something you all enjoy together.

You also need time for yourself. Make the most of it when it does come your way by putting all the 'shoulds' and 'oughts' completely out of your mind and concentrating on sheer self-indulgence. A snappy, stressed, wound-up parent is not what your child needs. When it all feels too much for you – and it will, at some point – take up some sort of stress reduction programme. It could be anything from a yoga class, a New Age CD, a warm bath with a glass of wine and the latest trashy novel, to a session on your exercise bike – it's whatever works for *you*.

Here are some favourite stress-busting tips.

- Close your eyes, drop your shoulders to release the tension in them, and spend a few moments breathing in . . . and out . . . very slowly.

- Make sure there's some greenery in your everyday life. It has been shown that walking under trees reduces blood pressure and that hospital patients recover more quickly if they can see trees through the ward window. Go for a walk in the park or along the riverbank. Treat yourself to a bunch of flowers or some easy-care house-plants. Grow your own veggies or herbs in pots.
- Relax by candlelight in the evening.
- Give yourself a spa treatment at home.
- Get your partner to give you a massage (you could return the favour!) or treat yourself to one at a local salon.
- Tune in to a different radio station from usual – Classic FM if you're a pop fan, Radio 2 instead of Radio 4.
- Take up a form of exercise particularly recommended for relaxation. As well as yoga, you could consider meditation, t'ai chi, Autogenic Training or something physical like Pilates or swimming.
- Contact with the natural world is proven to have a therapeutic effect – see the section on horse-riding. You might find walking the family dog or stroking the cat helps you to 'switch off'.
- Laugh! Dr Robert Holden, who set up the first Laughter Clinic in the UK, recommends what he calls 'transcendental chuckling', which means sitting in front of a mirror and laughing for two minutes for no reason at all . . .
- Take yourself to your favourite 'happy place'. There must be somewhere, some time, when you felt completely relaxed and at peace. It could be on a favourite holiday beach, in a chair by the fire, in your garden or even in bed. Close your eyes for five minutes and take yourself there. See it in your mind's eye, feel it, listen to the sounds of the sea, smell the crackle of burning logs, feel your cat's soft fur or your partner's arms round you. When you open your eyes again and come back to reality, the worst of your tension should have melted away.

# Useful addresses

There are a lot of organizations – some government sponsored, some charitable, some focused on self-help – which offer information and support to the parents of children with disabilities, including cerebral palsy. The popularity of the Internet has also led to the setting up of many online forums, often run by parents themselves.

**Advance Centre for The Scotson Technique:** tel.: 01342 311137; website: www.scotsontechnique.com

**Advisory Centre for Education:** helpline: 0808 800 5793; website: www .ace-ed.org.uk; help for parents of children aged 5–16 in State education, with information on special educational needs, bullying and exclusion

**Air Transport Users Council:** tel.: 020 7240 6061; website: www.auc.org .uk; information on hand-luggage restrictions and help for travellers with disabilities

**Alliance for Inclusive Education (ALLFIE):** tel.: 020 7737 6030; website: www.allfie.org.uk; organization campaigning for children with special needs to be educated in mainstream schools which are committed to removing all the barriers to full participation

**Assist UK:** tel.: 0870 770 2866; website: www.assist-uk.org; network of Disabled Living Centres where you can try equipment

**Benefits Enquiry Line:** tel.: 0800 882 200

**Bliss:** Family Support Helpline: 0500 618 140; website: www.bliss.org.uk; charity campaigning on behalf of premature babies

**Bobath Centre:** tel.: 020 8444 3355; website: www.bobath.org.uk

**Break:** tel.: 01263 822161; website: www.break-charity.org; low-cost holidays for families with disabled children

**Brook:** helpline: 0808 802 1234; website: www.brook.org.uk; confidential help with sex and relationships education for young people

**Carers UK:** helpline: 0808 808 7777; website: www.carersuk.org

**Center Parcs:** tel.: 08448 267723; website: www.centerparcs.co.uk; information on which activities are suitable for disabled guests

**Cerebra:** helpline: 0800 328 1159; website: www.cerebra.org.uk; help for parents of children with brain-related disorders; also funds research and gives grants

**Cerebral Palsy Physiotherapy Centre:** tel.: 01525 718581; website: www .cppcltd.co.uk

**Challenging Behaviour Foundation:** Family Support Line: 0845 602 7885; website: www.challengingbehaviour.org.uk

**Childline:** helpline: 0800 1111; for children in distress

**Citizens Advice:** website: www.citizensadvice.org.uk

**Contact a Family:** helpline: 0808 808 3555; website: www.cafamily.org.uk; puts parents of children with disabilities in touch with one another

**Crossroads Caring for Carers:** tel.: 0845 450 0350; website: www.crossroads .org.uk (England and Wales), www.crossroads-scotland.co.uk (Scotland), www.crossroadscare.co.uk (N. Ireland)

**Department for Children, Schools and Families Publications:** tel.: 0845 602 2260; website: publications.dcsf.gov.uk; for the *SEN: A guide for parents and carers* and *Direct Payments* booklets

**Department for Work and Pensions:** website: www.dwp.gov.uk

**Disability Law Service:** tel.: 020 7791 9800; website: www.dls.org.uk

**Disability Living Allowance:** Disability Benefits Helpline: 08457 123456; website: www.direct.gov.uk

**Disabled Living Foundation:** helpline: 0845 130 9177; website: www.dlf .org.uk; gives advice on equipment and mobility products

**DVLA:** tel.: 0870 240 0010; for information about road tax exemption for disabled people

**Elizabeth Finn Care:** tel.: 0800 413 200; website: www.elizabethfinncare .org.uk; grants for low-income families in need

**Enable Holidays:** tel.: 0871 222 4939; website: www.enableholidays.com; for information about holidays in Europe and the USA for people with disabilities

**Equality and Human Rights Commission:** helpline: 0845 604 6610 (England), 0845 604 5510 (Scotland), 0845 604 8810 (Wales)

**ERIC (Education and Resources for Improving Childhood Continence):** tel.: 0845 370 8008; website: www.eric.org.uk; help with incontinence in children

**Family Fund:** tel.: 0845 130 4542; website: www.familyfundtrust.org.uk; gives grants to low-income families with disabled children

**The Foundation for Conductive Education:** tel.: 0121 449 1569; website: www.conductive-education.org.uk

**FPA:** helpline: 0845 122 8690 (England and Wales), 0845 122 8687 (Northern Ireland); website: www.fpa.org.uk; help with sex and relationships education

**FRANK:** National Drugs Helpline: 0800 776600; website: www.talktofrank .com; confidential 24-hour information and help on drugs issues

**Hearing and Mobility:** tel.: 0844 888 1338; website: www.hearingand mobility.co.uk; company selling aids to daily living including mobility and incontinence aids

**HM Revenue and Customs:** Charities helpline: 0845 302 0203; website: www.hmrc.gov.uk; information on VAT reductions for people with disabilities

**ICAN:** tel.: 0845 225 4071; website: www.ican.org.uk; campaigns on behalf of those with communication difficulties

**IPSEA (Independent Panel for Special Education Advice):** helpline: 0800 018 4016; website: www.ipsea.org.uk

**KIDS:** tel.: 020 7520 0405; website: www.kids.org.uk; community projects in various parts of the UK which include children with disabilities

**Kidscape:** parents' anti-bullying helpline: 08451 205 204

**La Leche League:** helpline: 0845 120 2918; website: www.laleche.org.uk; advice on breastfeeding

**Motability:** tel.: 0845 456 4566; website: www.motability.co.uk; information on adapted cars

**National Childbirth Trust:** helpline: 0300 33 00 770 (enquiries); website: www.nct.org.uk; information on pregnancy, birth and baby care

**National Childminding Association:** helpline: 0800 169 4486; website: www.ncma.org.uk; has national networks catering for children with disabilities

**National Parent Partnership Network:** tel.: 020 7843 6058; website: www.parentpartnership.org.uk; details of local parent partnership services offering advice to parents of children with special needs

**National Portage Association:** website: www.portage.org.uk; early-years home-based education for children with special needs

**The National Society for Epilepsy:** helpline: 01494 601400; website: www.epilepsysociety.org.uk

**NHS Stop Smoking helpline:** tel.: 0800 169 0169

**Norman Laud Association:** tel.: 0121 373 6860; website: www.normanlaud .org.uk; provides day and respite care services in the West Midlands

**Outsiders:** sex and disability helpline: 07074 993 527; website www .outsiders.org.uk; friendship and social club for disabled over–16s

**Parentline Plus:** helpline: 0808 800 2222; website: www.parentlineplus .org.uk; help with all parenting issues

**Parents for Inclusion:** helpline: 0800 652 3145; website: www.parents forinclusion.org; campaigns for the rights of special-needs children in mainstream schools

**Pension Service:** tel.: 0845 606 0265; website: www.thepensionservice.gov .uk; for a booklet on pensions for carers

**PINNT (Patients on Intravenous and Naso-Gastric Nutrition Therapy):** tel.: 01202 481625; website: www.pinnt.co.uk

**Positive Parenting:** tel.: 0845 643 1939; website: www.parenting.org.uk; runs courses and workshops for parents including parents of special-needs children

**Pre-School Learning Alliance:** tel.: 020 7697 2500; website: www .pre-school.org.uk; information on playgroups and nurseries for children with special needs

**Princess Royal Trust for Carers:** tel.: 0844 800 4361; website: www.carers .org

**Riding for the Disabled Association:** tel.: 0845 658 1082; website: www .riding-for-disabled.org.uk

**SCOPE:** helpline (SCOPE Response): 0808 800 3333; website: www.scope .org.uk; the main campaigning group for people with cerebral palsy and their families

**Second Skin:** tel.: 0131 449 9497; website: www.secondskin.com.au; information about Lycra Dynamic Splinting

**Shared Care Network:** tel.: 0117 941 5361; website: www.sharedcarenetwork .org.uk

**TAMBA:** helpline: 0800 138 0509; website: www.tamba.org.uk; information and support for parents of twins, triplets and more

**Tommy's:** 'Ask our midwives' helpline: 0870 777 3060; website: www .tommys.org; charity for pregnant women and babies offering free leaflets on healthy pregnancy

**Tourism for All:** tel.: 0845 124 9971; website: www.tourismforall.org.uk; information on UK holidays for families with disabled children

**Traveline:** tel.: 0871 200 2233; website: www.traveline.info; information about accessible public transport in the UK

**Vitalise:** tel.: 0845 345 1972; website: www.vitalise.org.uk; runs holidays in the UK for families with disabled children, teenagers and adults

**Whizz-Kidz:** tel.: 020 7233 6600; website: www.whizz-kidz.org.uk; children's charity providing mobility aids

**Young Minds:** parents' helpline: 0808 802 5544; website: www.youngminds .org.uk; help with young people's emotional problems

## Other useful websites

**www.actionforkids.org:** help in removing barriers to independence

**www.adviceguide.org.uk:** information on benefits etc. from Citizens Advice

**www.direct.gov.uk:** information for carers on money, rights, assessments etc.

**www.disabilityalliance.org:** fact sheets and information on disability benefits

**www.earlysupport.org.uk:** a government programme to improve support for the families of young children with disabilities

**www.edcm.org.uk:** information about the Every Disabled Child Matters campaign for equal rights countrywide

**www.forparentsbyparents.com:** an A–Z of helpful organisations including those for children with special needs

**www.handyhealthcare.co.uk:** equipment, wheelchairs and toys for children with special needs

**www.hemihelp.org.uk:** support for families where a member has one-sided weakness

**www.makingcontact.org:** linking families with disabled children

**www.newlifecharity.co.uk:** equipment, wheelchairs and toys for children with special needs

**www.nhs.uk/carersdirect:** information for carers

**www.specialkidsintheuk.org:** parents' support group

**www.special-needs-kids.co.uk:** information directory and shopping site

**www.twin2twin.org:** for children with Twin to Twin Transfusion Syndrome (TTTS) and their parents

**ukfamily.co.uk:** includes examples of the kind of questions you might ask a SENCO or head teacher

**www.youngcarers.net:** support for young carers

**www.youreable.com:** practical information on issues like transport

# Index